AF560295

Innovations in Dairy Sciences

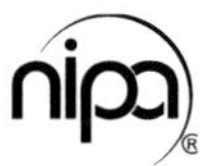

NIPA® GENX ELECTRONIC RESOURCES & SOLUTIONS P. LTD.

New Delhi-110 034

Abouth the Editors

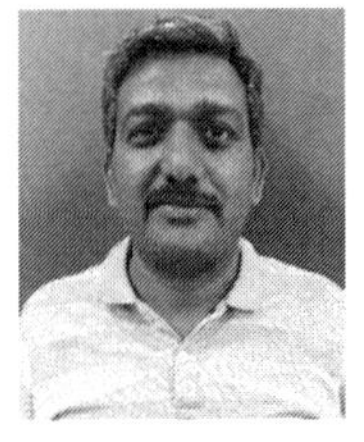

Manishkumar Parmar, [B.Tech. (D.T.), MBA (Marketing Management)] is working as an Assistant Professor, Dairy Business Management Department, College of Dairy Science, Kamdhenu University, Gujarat Since 2010 to present date. Having more than 12 years of experience in academic field and about 4 years expertise in dairy industry. He has published 06 research papers in various journals. He has also published book chapters, popular articles, vernaculars articles etc. His expertise to educate trained and motivate milk producer/ farmer through various extension activities via demonstration, radio talk, TV shows etc.

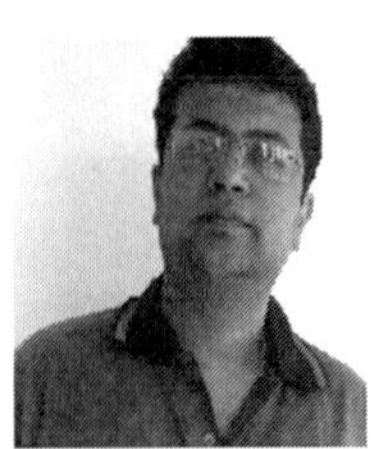

Tanmay Hazra, completed Ph.D. in Dairy Chemistry from NDRI, Karnal. He was awarded ICAR- SRF and Institute fellowship during pursuing Ph.D. He has published more than 22 research papers in various national and international journals; he also published 35 technical articles in different renowned magazines. He has received various awards including best paper award, young scientist award and young researchers from different scientific societies. Since 2016 he is working as an Assistant Professor in Kamdhenu University, Gujarat. He has completed 05 research projects from various funding agencies with one recommendation from AGRESCO. He also guided 06 M.Tech students.

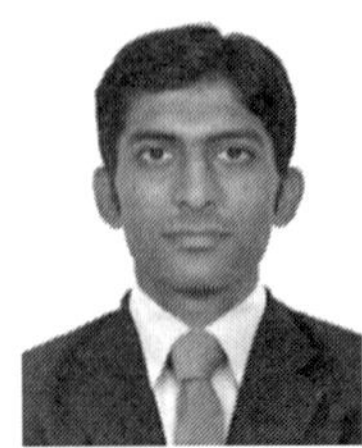

Rohit G. Sindhav completed B.Tech and M.Tech in Dairy Technology from SMC College of Dairy Science, Anand Agricultural University, Anand, Gujarat. Presently he is working as an Assistant Professor at College of Dairy Science, Kamdhenu University, Amreli, Gujarat. He has published 08 research papers in various national & international journals. He has also published book, book chapters and popular articles.

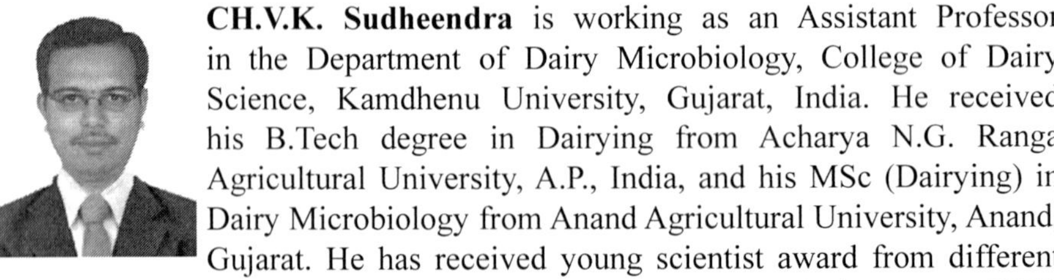

CH.V.K. Sudheendra is working as an Assistant Professor in the Department of Dairy Microbiology, College of Dairy Science, Kamdhenu University, Gujarat, India. He received his B.Tech degree in Dairying from Acharya N.G. Ranga Agricultural University, A.P., India, and his MSc (Dairying) in Dairy Microbiology from Anand Agricultural University, Anand, Gujarat. He has received young scientist award from different scientific societies. He is a life member of various scientific societies: IDA; AFSTI; AMI; SASNET-Fermented Foods. He has published several book chapters, research, review, and popular articles in national and international journals.

Innovations in Dairy Sciences

Manishkumar Parmar
Assistant Professor
Dairy Business Management Department
College of Dairy Science
Kamdhenu University, Gujarat

Tanmay Hazra
Assistant Professor
Department of Dairy Chemistry
College of Dairy Science
Kamdhenu University
Gujarat, India.

Rohit G. Sindhav
Assistant Professor
Department of Dairy Technology
College of Dairy Science
Kamdhenu University
Gujarat, India

CH.V.K. Sudheendra
Assistant Professor
Department of Dairy Microbiology
College of Dairy Science
Kamdhenu University
Gujarat, India

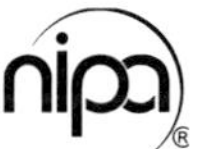

NIPA® GENX ELECTRONIC RESOURCES & SOLUTIONS P. LTD.
New Delhi-110 034

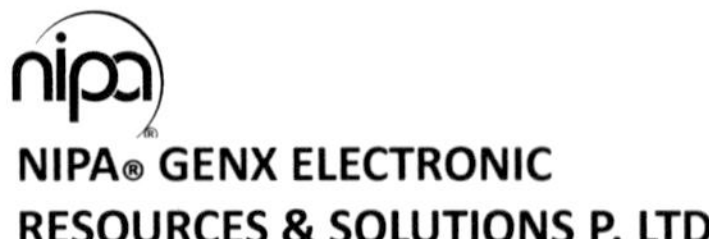

NIPA® GENX ELECTRONIC RESOURCES & SOLUTIONS P. LTD.

101,103, Vikas Surya Plaza, CU Block
L.S.C. Market, Pitam Pura, New Delhi-110 034
Ph : +91 11 27341616, 27341717, 27341718
E-mail: newindiapublishingagency@gmail.com
Website: www.nipabooks.com

For customer assistance, please contact
Phone: + 91-11-27 34 17 17
Fax: + 91-11-27 34 16 16
E-Mail: feedbacks@nipabooks.com

ISBN: 978-81-19103-22-5

Composed and Designed by NIPA®.

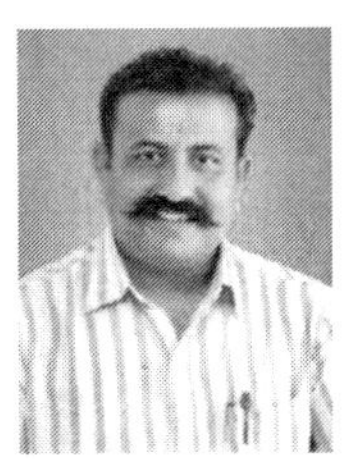

Ashvin Savaliya
Chairman, AMR Dairy, Amreli

Message

The wholesomeness of milk as a complete functional food is recognized whole world today, especially in this tough COVID- 19 pandemic situation. The whole world's medical fraternity emphasized the personal immunity for fighting against Corona virus. In such a situation, apan from medicine or vaccination, the role of immune boosting foods has been proved very efficient for the treatment of COVID patients. Milk is an ample source of different immune boosting bioactive components like immunoglobulin, lactoferrin, lysozome, different growth factor s, essential fatty acids etc. Some in-vitro studies suggested that milk derived lactoferrin is very effective against SARS — COVID- virus.

Indian dairy culture are always pioneering to the world. Lord Krishna can be considered the first recognized dairy personnel and pioneer of organized dairy farming. From Post impendence era the growth of milk producing is increasing continuously and India is the largest milk producing country throughout the world; producing almost 198MMT of milk in the year 2020-21. Indian dairy industry is mainly accompanied by un-organized sector but post White revolution and formation of AMUL organization pattern change the scenario of whole Indian dairy Industry. AMUL organization pattern able to organize more than 36 Lakhs dairy farmers. Dairy industry are now these days contributing the largest portion of Indian agriculture GDP. Consequent to the Union Budget 2017-18 announcement, Dairy Processing & Infrastructure Development Fund has been set up with a corpus of Rs. 8,004 crore with National Bank for Agriculture and Rural Development (NABARD).

AMR Dairy is the district co-operative of Amreli, Gujarat and our main motto is the development of dairy farmers associated with dairy farming. So, we always encourage the innovations in dairy industry. The Book on the recent development of Milk and Dairy Industry shall be a very good insight for the Industry to increase the horizons of Dairy Industry.

I wish all success to the Authors and Editors.

Ashvin Savaliya
Chairman, AMR Dairy, Amreli

Preface

Milk is nature's perfect food; recommended to all age groups for a healthy body. Developing countries are facing scarcity of milk especially in urban areas. This may be due to the factors like lack of processing facilities and application of advanced processing methodologies. In recent times dramatic changes have taken place in dairy industry by adopting latest technologies. New technologies are emerging with advancement of scientific knowledge in dairying. At present there are books on various processing techniques, quality control methods, but are scattered across several books. Hence, the editors envisaged an idea to bring together all the advanced processing techniques, quality control methods and various applications into an abridged book in simplified language which can be easily understood by entrepreneurs, academicians, researchers researchers, farmers, and industrialists and keep them abreast with latest technologies.

The contributions by the cooperating authors to this book have been the most valuable in the compilation. Their names are mentioned in each chapter. This book would not have been written without their valuable cooperation, many of whom are renowned scientists as well as talented researchers in the field of dairying.

This book is compiled of eleven chapters, divided into three categories. First category is dedicated to processing techniques starting with a brief introduction of all the latest processing technologies in chapter 1, followed by chapters on High pressure processing, Pulsed electric field technology, cold plasma technology. Second category comprises of quality aspects in chapter 5 on aptamers, followed by microbial biosensors, FTIR spectroscopy, Nano Science in Dairy Quality. Finally third part comprises of application part with Enzyme Based Flavour Components, Applications of modified starch, Nutrigenomics.

We would like to thank Publisher NIPA (New India Publishing Agency), for making every effort to publish the book when milk issues are major issues worldwide. Special thanks are also due to the NIPA Production Staff. I request that readers to offer their constructive suggestions that may help us to improve the next edition.

We express our deep sense of gratitude to our families for their continuos understanding, cooperation and love during the preparation of the book..

Editors

Contents

1

Alternative (Eco-friendly) Milk Processing Systems

Kuntal Roy[1*], Partha Pratim Debnath[1], Anindita Debnath[1] Ronit Mandal[2] and Payal Karmakar[3]

[1]Assistant Professor, Department of Dairy Technology, West Bengal University of Animal and Fishery Sciences (WBUAFS), PO Krishi Viswa Vidyalaya, Mohanpur, 741252, West Bengal, India
[2]Faculty of Land and Food Systems, University of British Columbia, Vancouver, BC V6T 1Z4, Canada
[3]Dairy Chemistry Division, NDRI, Karnal - 132001 Haryana, India

Abstract

Now a days people prefer less processed, highly nutritious food with no added preservatives. These compels food sectors to develop modern methods of processing to fulfill the demand of consumers. Milk is perishable, and for this reason, it needs to be processed to increase its shelf life. Traditionally, milk is processed by high temperature processing such as pasteurization, sterilization to improve its shelf life. However, the application of high temperature causes changes in the structural and functional properties of milk components as well as decrease in the nutritional value. It is possible to keep the inherent properties of milk intact along with microbial destruction through application of nonthermal processes. The Non-thermal technological processes include high pressure processing, pulsed electric field, radio frequency processing, pulsed UV light processing, bactofugation, ultrasound processing, irradiation, cold plasma, ozone treatment and membrane technology (microfiltration). In this chapter, the above mentioned alternate methods which are eco-friendly, are discussed.

Introduction

Milk is considered to be a perfect food which contains almost all the macro- and micronutrients required for normal body growth. However, it is highly perishable in nature which poses problem during its storage. It gets spoiled within few hours after milking if not processed or cooled immediately. It can also be a source of several disease causing microbes as it is conducive for the growth of microorganisms.

Food preservation is a method of maintaining desired food quality and safety as long as possible by minimizing the rate of quality deterioration as well as microbial proliferation. Therefore, the study on the impact of the preservation processes on the quality attributes on top of safety aspects of food is important. Traditionally milk is thermally processed by processes such as pasteurization, sterilization, ultra-high heat (UHT) treatment, concentration and drying. Many of these processes decrease the nutritional value of milk or may cause adverse effects on the sensory properties. Now a days the consumers demand fresh and natural food, free from chemical preservatives and other harmful additives, which are minimally heat processed, and at the same time also have a reasonable shelf life with assured quality. Nonthermal methods can be applied as an alternative to traditional themal processing methods for controlling microorganisms, inactivating enzymes, retaining the sensory properties and nutritional value of milk. These processes are called non thermal methods as they do not raise the temperature of the products significantly. In this chapter, the nonthermal processes like high pressure processing, pulsed electric field, radio frequency processing, pulsed UV light processing, bactofugation, ultrasound processing, irradiation, cold plasma, ozone treatment and microfiltration, are discussed with respect to milk processing.

High Pressure Processing

High-pressure processing (HPP) is an emerging nonthermal food processing technology. In this technique, the intense hydrostatic pressure is used instead of temperature to inactivate spoilage causing as well as pathogenic microorganisms. The pressure applied is between 100 and 800 MPa to packaged and non-packaged foods. The treated products are reported to be safe, and have better texture with extended shelf life. It also increases the retention of nutrients in comparison to thermally processed foods.

HPP operation depends on three basic principles that are used to explain its working (Mandal and Kant, 2017). These are Le-Chatelier's principle, Pascal's isostatic principle and principle of microscopic ordering. According to Le-Chatelier's principle, "a system always tries to act to resist changes in chemical equilibrium. To restabilize the equilibrium the system will favour a chemical pathway that will reduce disturbance. The reactions that result in the reduced volume, enhanced under high pressure" result in the inactivation of microorganisms or enzymes. The isostatic principle states that "when a food product is under pressure, then the pressure acts uniformly in all directions." As per microscopic ordering principle "at a constant temperature an increase in pressure increases the degrees of the molecule ordering. Therefore, temperature and pressure exert opposing forces on molecular structure and chemical reactions."

Application of HHP causes remarkable change in cell structure such as destruction of intracellular vacuoles, separation of cell-wall and cytoplasmic membrane, leakage of intracellular components, destruction of the ribosome and loss of homeostasis. These damages in the cell morphology cause the loss of cell functions, lowering of growth rate and even cell lysis. HHP treatment also causes an increase in the level of extracellular ATP and transport of ethidium bromide and propidium iodide to cell, indication of the loss of membrane permeability and function. It was noticed that gram-positive bacteria are more resistant to HPP than gram-negative bacteria (Mandal and Kant, 2017). An application of 500–600 MPa at 25°C for 10 min is required to inactivate gram-positive microorganisms. Whereas, gram-negative microorganisms require relatively low pressures under the same temperature-time combination to get inactivated (Smelt, 1998). The inactivation of virus by HPP is due to the denaturation of capsid proteins. In terms of the microbiological quality of milk, HPP at 400–600 MPa is comparable to that of pasteurized milk (Buffa *et al.*, 2000). But due to the resistance of spores to high pressure, it is not comparable to sterilized milk. Rademacher and Kessler (1997) suggested the application of HPP of either 400 MPa for 15 min or 600 MPa for 3 min at 20°C to milk, to get a shelf-life of 10 days at 10°C.

The application of 100-600 MPa leads to an increase in the ionic calcium, phosphate and magnesium in milk serum. Merel-Rausch (2007) noticed a little effect on the changes in casein micelle sizes at a pressure of 100–200 MPa at room temperature, whereas at a pressure higher than 300 MPa, the size of casein micelle almost reduced to half. HPP processing of milk has also caused a reduction in the size of the fat globule, denaturation of whey proteins and inactivation of some enzymes such as plasmin. Most of the milk enzymes loss its activity at a pressure above 300 MPa. HPP is also shown to preserve bovine colostrum after 400 MPa treatment for 20 min (Foster *et al.*, 2016).

Pulsed Electric Field

Pulsed Electric Field (PEF) is another nonthermal process, which can be used in place of the conventional thermal methods to inactivate the microorganisms as well as enzymes. PEF can be only applied for a pumpable foods such as milk and juices, however, its application in drying and extraction encompasses solid products too. This process does not significantly increase the temperature of the product nor even changes the food properties such as color, odour, taste, protein and vitamin C contents. The mechanism of PEF process involves the application of short pulses of high-intensity electric field. The liquid flows between two electrodes for a few milliseconds and achieve the desired inactivation of microbial load. Generally, 20-80 kV/cm of multiple short-duration pulses are applied for less than a few micro seconds. Electroporation and cellular leakage are the two most accepted principles responsible for microbial inactivation. The electroporation theory involves destruction of the microbial cell by disruption of its membrane. The application of a high voltage electrical field causes enlargement of the microbial pores on the cell membrane, which causes the release of cellular constituents into the medium (Wiktor *et al.,* 2020). During the process, some stable hydrophobic pores are produced, which can conduct electric current without causing localized heating effects. The proteins of the cell membrane get destabilized and lipid bilayer of membrane converted to crystalline lipid from a rigid gel structure. Thus, the cell plasma membrane becomes more permeable causes entry of foreign molecules into the cell results in swelling and disintegration of the cell membrane (Garcia *et al.,* 2007). According to the electrical breakdown theory, the bacterial cell membrane act as a capacitor filled with the dielectric material of low electric conductance and a dielectric constant of 2. The potential difference (PD) across the membrane is about 10 mV. The PD increased when subjected to an external electric field. The increase in PD reduces the thickness of the membrane. Larger pores are formed in the membrane when the PD across the cell membrane reaches a critical level of about 1 V. Formation of large pores causes discharge of cell material and further damage of the membrane (Zimmermann, 1986).

It was examined that PEF application is effective on microorganisms such as *Staphylococcus aureus*, *Escherichia coli*, *Bacillus subtilis, Listeria monocytogenes, Bacillus cereus* and *Saccharomyces cerevisiae*. Numerous researchers worked to evaluate the effect of different intensities of PEF in the inactivation of various microorganisms in milk. Raso *et al.* (1999) reduced the microbial count by 2 $\log_{10}$ in raw skimmed milk after PEF application. In UHT milk, the 3 $\log_{10}$ reduction of *Bacillus stearothermophilus* was observed after application of 60 kV/cm electric field at 50 °C for 210 µs (Shin *et al.,* 2007).

PEF treated milk has shelf life of more than 14 days at refrigerated condition. PEF treatment was reported to have the ability to inactivate many enzymes. Partial unfolding of proteins, destabilization of electrostatic regions in the structure by external electric fields, oxidation-reduction reactions supposedly cause inactivation of enzymes. A 65% reduction of alkaline phosphatase in skimmed milk and 59% in whole milk was observed, during the application of PEF at 18.8 kV/cm electric field force at 70 pulses (Castro *et al.,* 2001). No significant change in color, pH, particle size, conductivity, total solids and protein content was observed in PEF treated UHT skim milk (Michalac *et al.,* 2003). The effect of PEF processing in the range from 1.8 to 2.7 kV/mm of electric field on vitamins showed that about 90% of vitamin C retained and other vitamins remained unaltered. At field strengths of 80 kV/cm, fat and protein integrity was not affected (Deeth *et al.,* 2007). The application of PEF technology has been restricted to select microbes in milk, as the effect of PEF on the physical and chemical constituents of milk are yet not fully understood. Also, with the advancement in the design and development of PEF systems, it is expected that economic and cost-effective equipment would lead to wider adoption of the technology on a commercial scale.

Radio Frequency Processing

Radio frequency electric field (RFEF) heating is another nonthermal process where the power supply is in continuous form, unlike PEF, with frequency ranging from 3 kHz to 300 GHz. The frequency for industrial, scientific, and medical use are 13.56 MHz, 27.12 MHz and 40.68 MHz, respectively. The chief benefit of this method is the rapid and volumetric development of heat inside the product, which causes uniform heating in short times. RF waves have high penetration depth, which makes it suitable for pre-packed food products. RFEF at 30 kV/cm, 21 kHz reduced *E. coli* by 4.8 log at 60°C in apple cider, whereas conventional heating at the same conditions did not affect *E. coli* (Geveke and Brunkhorst, 2008). In general, commercial extended shelf-life milk subjected to heat treatments (120°C) has a shelf life of about 20–25 days, whereas the radio frequency heating process shows a shelf life of up to 55 days at 4°C (Di Rosa *et al.,* 2018).

Pulsed Ultraviolet Light

Electromagnetic radiation having a wavelength between X-ray and visible ray is known as ultraviolet (UV) radiation. These have a wavelength of 100 to 400 nm. UV radiation, because of its short wavelength and high energy, has the capability to inactivate several types of microorganisms. Pulsed UV light processing is a novel nonthermal process which involves application of high intensity pulses of light. It is used to disinfect the food or packaging surface decontamination. It maintains the texture and nutrients of the treated food. The mechanism of microbial inactivation by pulsed UV light is due to photothermal and photochemical methods (Mandal *et al.*, 2020). Due to photochemical mechanism, the UV light of germicidal wavelength 253.7 nm leads to dimer formation in DNA which leads to hinderances in cell replication and an eventual lysis. Above 300 nm the germicidal action decreases (Bachmann, 1975). UV light having 254 nm wavelength is generally used for the disinfection of water, food and surface of packaging material. The penetration capacity of UV light varies with the state of matter, that's why it has more germicidal activity in the liquid than solid foods. The penetration capacity even depends upon the level of solids dissolved in the liquid, whereby the transparent clear liquid shows more reduction in the microbial population (Mandal *et al.*, 2020). Both postive as well as negative reports could be found on the impact of pulsed UV light on milk and milk products. Pulsed UV light was shown inactivate the pathogenic organism *Staphylococcus aureus* in milk (Krishnamurthy *et al.*, 2010). Milk is photosensitive in nature and for this reason, off flavour developed in milk after application of UV light. It causes hydrolytic rancidity and oxidation of milk fat. However, no remarkable difference was noticed in the percentage of malondialdehyde and other reactive substances between treated and untreated milk. Processing of milk by UV light also causes loss of vitamin B2, vitamin A, vitamin C and E (Gunesar and Yuceer, 2012). Among individual effect of UV and pasteurization of raw milk, the latter is more effective than the former. But the efficiency can be increased by using in combination with other preservative techniques.

Bactofugation

Bactofugation is a nonthermal centrifugal process for removing microorganisms and spores of microorganisms from milk. During bactofugation, the milk is separated into two streams in a special centrifuge called bactofuge: milk and bactofugate. The bactofuge exerts a force of approximately 9,000 x g on the milk. Bactofugate consists of bacterial mass with density of 1.2 to 1.3 g/mL, which is denser than the milk and gets separated at a rate governed by Stokes' law. The bactofugate is 2-3% of the total input. Later the bactofugate is sterilized by direct steam injection at 140°C for 3-4 sec, cooled and re-mixed with the clarified milk. The entire process is carried out continuously in a Bactotherm line. Bactofugation removes 98% of anaerobic spore-forming organisms and 95% of aerobic spore formers from the milk. It can reduce the total count of bacteria by 86% of milk. Milk psychrotrophs are responsible for milk deterioration. They produce lipases and proteases, which significantly reduce the quality and shelf life of processed milk. In a study by Junior *et al.* (2019), preheating of milk caused the elimination of 99.99% of psychotropic bacteria, while bactofugation further reduced 89.66% of psychrotrophs from the preheated milk. This process maintains the milk nutritional and functional properties. It is highly suitable for processing milk for cheese, and other products.

Ultrasonication

Ultrasound is high-intensity longitudinal sound waves that can cause acoustic streaming and cavitation. This phenomenon leads to numerous changes in the functional characteristics of food. The practical application of ultrasonication nowadays has become very common as it is a fast, versatile and nonthermal process. Application of ultrasound is usually within the frequencies of 20 kHz to 10 Mhz. It can propagate through solid, liquid and gas. In the liquid phase, the propagation of the wave causes the formation of alternating compression and expansion cycles. The rapid, continuous and successive expansion and compression causes a change in pressure and as a consequence forms small air bubbles. These bubbles progressively coalesce with each other, increases in size and volume. On attaining a threshold figure, the bubbles collapse due to its inability to absorb further energy. The cycle of formation, expansion and collapsing of air bubbles is known as cavitation. The collapse of air bubbles generates shock waves with local heat (approximately 5000 K) and pressure (50000 kPa). These localized pressure and temperature fluctuations results in cell disruption and a localized sterilization effect. Complete inactivation of microorganisms and enzymes requires longer treatment time, which causes an increase in energy consumption. Numerous researches were carried out on the ultrasonication in milk, which showed negligible adverse effects as compared with conventional heat treatment. Ultrasound serves many other functions other than the bactericidal effect and inactivation of the enzyme. Ultrasound is also used for homogenization of milk fat and degassing in the milk. It even improves the structural as well as the functional properties of dairy ingredients, and ultrasound can enhance the antioxidant activity of fermented milk. The application of ultrasound at 20 kHz on milk fat globule showed a significant decrease in the size of fat globules up to 81.5% at room temperature. Cameron *et al.* (2009) noticed that the application of ultrasound (20 kHz) on milk for 10 min reduced *E. coli* and *L. monocytogenes* count by 100 and 99%, respectively. Ultrasound does not inactivate the alkaline phosphatase and lactoperoxidase activities.

Irradiation

Irradiation technology demonstrated great success in destroying various pathogenic and spoilage causing microorganisms. Irradiation includes the use of X-rays, accelerated electron beams and gamma rays as the sources of ionizing radiation for the preservation of food products. Generally gamma rays are produced by radioactive isotopes of ^{137}Cs and ^{60}Co. A highly energized electron or ray, when passes through food, penetrates through the bacteria cells, causing cell lysis by knocking out electrons from biomolecules. Milk treated with gamma radiation at 2.5 kGy shows a reduction in the total bacterial count by 98.98% and spore formers by 95.77% (Baky *et al.,* 1986). But the extension of the shelf life of dairy products using irradiation treatment is not a widely accepted system as it causes the formation of radiolytic products. It generates unacceptable off-odours and flavor via oxidation. Dairy products exposed to irradiation at a dose of 40 kGy at -78°C in the nitrogen-modified atmosphere resulted in little change in color or texture but caused the formation of off-flavor and after taste, which decreased the overall acceptability and characteristic flavour. Low dose irradiation did not affect the proximate compositions of various cheese products and color, pH, lactose and lactic acid content of plain yogurt. Therefore, irradiation with a low dose in combination with other freezing or modified atmospheric packaging or with preservatives such as sorbic acid can increase the shelf life without decreasing the quality.

Cold Plasma

Plasma is the fourth state of matter and known as quasi-neutral gas (Langmuir, 1928). When the gaseous state is given sufficiently high energy the plasma state occurs. It has a net charge zero as it is a mixture of both positive and negative charge particles. Plasma is an ionized gas that has many species like positive and negative ions, electrons, gas atoms, free electrons, free radicals, activated neutral species and quanta of electromagnetic radiation or photons (Mandal *et al.,* 2018). The phase transition from gaseous state to plasma state is accomplished by applying high kinetic energy to gaseous medium, which breaks intramolecular and intraatomic structure of gas and releases free electrons and ions. Energy sources such as mechanical, thermal, nuclear, radian or electric current are available for ionization of gas. Cold plasma also known as non- equilibrium plasma, nonthermal plasma has a low gas temperature and a high electron temperature (Mandal *et al.,* 2018).

The ability of plasma to inactivate a wide range of microorganisms including spores and viruses have been studied. When microbial cells are subjected to cold plasma the free radicals, reactive species, or charged particles of plasma accumulated at the surface of the cell membrane cause unrepairable surface lesion to living cell as well as perforation or cell leakage by lethal oxidation of unsaturated fatty acids of lipid bilayer of cell membrane, oxidation of amino acids and nucleic acid, denaturation of protein of cell membrane. In addition to reactive species, UV photons are known to modify DNA of microorganisms by dimerization and as a result disturb cell replication. Cold plasma technology has already been successfully applied for the surface sterilization of packaging material as well as modification of functional properties (Mandal *et al.*, 2018). This technology is in its infancy stage for decontamination of food and dairy products on the industrial scale. Tammineedi (2012) examined the effect of cold plasma on of *E. coli, S. aureus* and *S. Typhimurium* in whole, semi-skimmed and skimmed milk stored at 4°C for 42 days. It was observed that at 20 kV the counts of *E. coli*, *S. Typhimurium* and *S. aureus* were reduced to 3.63, 2.00 and 2.62 $\log_{10}$ CFU/mL, respectively. The application of plasma did not affect the pH and color. After one week of examination, no viable cells were detected in the whole milk that remained stable during storage.

Ozone Treatment

Ozone is a broad-spectrum powerful antimicrobial agent and is found to be active against bacteria, fungi, viruses, protozoa, and their spores. The germicidal action of ozonation is due to its capability to interact with cellular constituents – proteins, respiratory enzymes and unsaturated lipid. The ozone even interacts with the nucleic acids in the cytoplasm, proteins and peptidoglycan in spore coats, and virus capsids. Ozone is produced either by the exposure of air or a mixture of gas containing oxygen to an energy source such as a high-energy electrical field, UV radiation or through the conversion of O_2 to O_3. Ozone has a relatively inert effect on the sensory and nutritional quality of the product and that makes it advantageous over conventional antimicrobial agents. Previously ozone treatment was meant for only solid foods items either in the form of ozone gas or ozonated water. The treatment was mainly applied for surface decontamination of fruits and vegetables, wastewater treatment or drinking water disinfection. After approval from the United States Food and Drug Administration (FDA), the potential of ozonation in dairy applications has begun to exploit. Several researchers examined the application of ozone in milk and concluded that ozone treatment has the potential to be a nonthermal process for milk and milk products. Ozone is introduced into milk in a gaseous or aqueous state in a stirred-tank or bubble column reactor. A dose of 0.2 g/ h of ozone to raw milk for 15 min causes the elimination of *L. monocytogenes* with minimal impact on protein, carbohydrate, and calcium. Cavalcante *et al.* (2013) treated raw milk with ozone gas at 1.5 mg/L for 15 min. A significant reduction of Enterobacteriaceae, mesophilic aerobic, psychotropic bacteria, mold and yeast, and *Staphylococcus* by 0.96, 0.60, 0.13, 0.48 and 1.02 $\log_{10}$, respectively with respect to the amount of microorganism before ozonisation, was reported. Thus, for improving the microbial quality of raw milk ozonisation could be adopted as a pre-processing step.

Microfiltration

Membrane technology is another nonthermal process which has a high demand for its various application in the dairy sector. The application of membrane mainly depends upon the pore size of membrane and pressure applied for separation. Among all the other membrane separation, microfiltration (MF) is used for the reduction or separation of bacteria or spores from milk at lower temperature without hampering the nutritional quality of milk. MF can retain particles of size between 0.1 to 20 µm. This causes retention of fat globules, so for this reason, skim milk is used instead of whole milk for the MF process. A study by Pedersen (1992) showed that MF of skim milk can retain up to 99.10 to 99.90% of total bacteria. In this process spores of *Bacillus cereus* and other fermentative bacteria were retained more than 99.95% and 98.40%, respectively. Te Giffel and Horst (2004) reported that MF has the potential to separate more bacteria and spores as compared to bactofugation. It not only separates bacteria and spores but can increase the casein content of milk and can increase the sensorial quality of serum proteins. A combination of MF and thermal treatment increased the shelf life of milk to 33 days with minimal compositional change respect to the raw untreated milk (Garcia and Rodriguez 2014).

Conclusion

The emerging non-thermal technologies are energy-efficient processes to reduce the microbial load in milk without significantly altering its quality. The effectiveness of these processing technologies for microbial and enzyme inactivation within milk has been analyzed and correlated with traditional preservation methods by several researchers. But still, these methods are in their infancy. There is, however, a need for synchronization and comparison of data available from numerous researches to use these technologies at a commercial level. It is possible to use them in combination with other methods when they are not effective while used alone. Further research and development will help shape the path of their integration in the dairy industry.

References

Bachmann, R. (1975). Sterilization by intense ultraviolet-radiation. *Brown Boveri Review*, 62(5): 206-209.

Baky, A. A., Farahat, S. M., Rabie, A. M. & Mobasher, S. A. (1986). The manufacture of Ras cheese from gamma irradiated milk. *Food Chemistry*, 20(3): 201-212.

Buffa, M., Trujillo, A. J., Royo, C. & Guamis, B. (2000). Changes in chemical and microbiological characteristics of goat cheese made from raw, pasteurized or high-pressure-treated milk. *International Journal of High Pressure Research*, 19(1-6): 27-32.

Cameron, M., McMaster, L. D. & Britz, T. J. (2009). Impact of ultrasound on dairy spoilage microbes and milk components. *Dairy Science & Technology*, 89(1): 83-98.

Castro, A. J., Swanson, B. G., Barbosa-Canovas, G. V. & Meyer, R. (2001). Pulsed electric field modification of milk alkaline phosphatase activity. In *Pulsed Electric Fields in Food processing: Fundamental Aspects and Applications*, Technomic Publishing Company Inc., pp. 65-83.

Cavalcante, M. A., Leite Junior, B. R. C., Tribst, A. A. L. & Cristianini, M. (2013). Improvement of the raw milk microbiological quality by ozone treatment. *International Food Research Journal*, 20(4): 2017-2021.

Deeth, H. C., Datta, N., Ross, A. I. & Dam, X. T. (2007). Pulsed Electric Field Technology: Effect on Milk and Fruit Juices. In *Advances in thermal and non-thermal food preservation*, Blackwell Publishing, Iowa, USA, pp. 241-261.

Di Rosa, A. R., Leone, F., Bressan, F., Battaglia, G., Veccia, T. & Chiofalo, V. (2018). Radio frequency heating of milk–effects on quality, safety, and shelf life assessed using artificial senses and chemometric tools. *Electronics*, 7(12): 402.

Foster, D. M., Poulsen, K. P., Sylvester, H. J., Jacob, M. E., Casulli, K. E. & Farkas, B. E. (2016). Effect of high-pressure processing of bovine colostrum on immunoglobulin G concentration, pathogens, viscosity, and transfer of passive immunity to calves. *Journal of Dairy Science*, 99(11): 8575-8588.

Garcia, D., Gomez, N., Manas, P., Raso, J. & Pagan, R. (2007). Pulsed electric fields cause bacterial envelopes permeabilization depending on the treatment intensity, the treatment medium pH and the microorganism investigated. *International Journal of Food Microbiology*, 113(2): 219-227.

García, L. F. & Rodriguez, F. R. (2014). Combination of microfiltration and heat treatment for ESL milk production: Impact on shelf life. *Journal of Food Engineering*, 128: 1-9.

Geveke, D. J. & Brunkhorst, C. (2008). Radio frequency electric fields inactivation of Escherichia coli in apple cider. *Journal of Food Engineering*, 85(2): 215-221.

Guneser, O. & Yuceer, Y. K. (2012). Effect of ultraviolet light on water-and fat-soluble vitamins in cow and goat milk. *Journal of Dairy Science*, 95(11): 6230-6241.

Júnior, J. C. R., Peruzi, G. A., Bruzaroski, S. R., Tamanini, R., Lobo, C. M., Conti, A.C., Alfieri, A.A. & Beloti, V. (2019). Effect of bactofugation of raw milk on counts and microbial diversity of psychrotrophs. *Journal of Dairy Science*, 102(9): 7794-7799.

Langmuir, I. (1928). Oscillations in ionized gases. *Proceedings of the National Academy of Sciences of the United States of America*, 14(8): 627.

Mandal, R. & Kant, R. (2017). High-pressure processing and its applications in the dairy industry. *Food Science and Technology: An International Journal (FSTJ)*, 1(1): 33-45.

Mandal, R., Mohammadi, X., Wiktor, A., Singh, A. & Anubhav, P. S. (2020). Applications of Pulsed Light Decontamination Technology in Food Processing: An Overview. *Applied Sciences*, 10(10): 3606.

Mandal, R., Singh, A. & Singh, A. P. (2018). Recent developments in cold plasma decontamination technology in the food industry. *Trends in Food Science & Technology*, 80: 93-103.

Merel-Rausch, E. (2007). Hydrostatic high pressure treatment of casein to generate defined particle and gel structures. Doctoral Thesis. Fakultät Naturwissenschaften Universität Hohenheim.

Michalac, S., Alvarez, V.T.J.I., Ji, T. & Zhang, Q. H. (2003). Inactivation of selected microorganisms and properties of pulsed electric field processed milk. *Journal of Food Processing and Preservation*, 27(2): 137-151.

Pedersen, P. J. (1992). Microfiltration for the reduction of bacteria in milk and brine. *Bulletin-International Dairy Federation*, (1): 33-50.

Rademacher, B. & Kessler, H. G. (1997). High pressure inactivation of microorganisms and enzymes in milk and milk products. *High Pressure Research in Biosciences and Biotechnology*, Elsevier, Amsterdam, Netherland, pp. 291-293.

Raso, J., Gongora, M. M., Calderon, M. L., Barbosa-Canovas, G. V. & Swanson, B. G. (1999). Resistant microorganisms to high intensity pulsed electric field pasteurization of raw skim milk. In *IFT annual meeting technical program.*

Shin, J. K., Jung, K. J., Pyun, Y. R. & Chung, M. S. (2007). Application of Pulsed Electric Fields with Square Wave Pulse to Milk Inoculated with *E. coli*, *P. fluorescens*, and *B. stearothermophilus*. *Food Science and Biotechnology*, 16(6): 1082-1084.

Smelt, J. P. P. M. (1998). Recent advances in the microbiology of high pressure processing. *Trends in Food Science & Technology*, 9(4): 152-158.

Tammineedi, C.V.R.K. (2012). Effect of UV-C light, high intensity ultrasound and nonthermal atmospheric plasma treatments on the allergenity of major cow milk proteins. Master's Thesis, Southern Illinois University.

Te Giffel, M. C. & Van Der Horst, H. C. (2004). Comparison between bactofugation and microfiltration regarding efficiency of somatic cell and bacteria removal. *Bulletin-International Dairy Federation*, (389): 49-53.

Wiktor, A., Singh, A. P., Parniakov, O., Mykhailyk, V., Mandal, R. & Witrowa-Rajchert, D. (2020). PEF as an alternative tool to prevent thermolabile compound degradation during dehydration processes. In *Pulsed Electric Fields to Obtain Healthier and Sustainable Food for Tomorrow*. Academic Press, London, UK, pp. 155-202.

Zimmermann, U. (1986). Electrical breakdown, electropermeabilization and electrofusion. In *Reviews of Physiology, Biochemistry and Pharmacology,* Springer, Berlin, Germany, pp. 175-256.

2

High-Pressure Processing Novel Technology in Dairy Industry

Subhash Prasad and Kunalkumar Ahuja

Assistant Professor, College of Dairy Science, Amreli, Kamdhenu University Gandhinagar, Gujarat, India

Abstract

High-pressure processing (HPP) is a novel and non-thermal processing technology. Processing of foods by this method offers an alternative to thermal processing as it is carried out near the ambient temperature, thus, eliminating the adverse effects of heat and keeps the sensory and nutritional attributes of the food fresh like. Principal hindrances to adoption is the high cost of equipment and low throughput of HPP equipment, meaning high value, perishable materials are treated. This chapter outlines the salient principles of the high pressure processing, microbial inactivation effects, applications of high pressure in the processing of dairy products, effect of pressure treatment on the milk constituents, new trends and issues and challenge related adaptation of the HPP process in the dairy industry.

Introduction

High-pressure processing (HPP) is a novel method for non-thermal preservation technique of food that inactivates harmful pathogens and vegetative spoilage microorganisms. HPP is an alternate, non-thermal food processing method, wherein the food is subjected to a very high pressure range from 100 -800 MPa (1MPa = 145.03 Psi or 10 Bar). HPP is also referred as High hydrostatic pressure processing, Ultra high-pressure processing, Hyperbaric processing and Pascalization (Rao *et al.,* 2014). Theoretically pressure-temperature operational conditions for HPP treatment of foods may range from 100 to 800 MPa at -20°C to 121°C, depending on the process and the nature of the food. It allows to be pasteurization of milk at or near room temperature.

In HPP, small molecules, which are the characteristics of flavouring and nutritional components, typically remain unchanged by pressure (Horie *et al.*, 1991). HPP processed foods have better texture and colour compared to that of heat processed foods. This technique improves food safety by destroying the bacteria that can cause food borne illness and spoilage, but the food remains fresh. HPP as a clean label technology has found a growing acceptance in the dairy and food industries for producing high-quality foods.

Application of HPP for milk preservation began when (Hite, 1899) demonstrated that the shelf life of milk could be extended. The first commercial HP-treated products (high acid jam) appeared on the market in 1991 in Japan.HPP is now being used for products such as dairy foods, fruit juices, jams, sauces, rice, cakes and desserts etc. (Tao *et al.*, 2014; Muntean *et al.*, 2016). Recent studies have focused on the effects of HPP on health attributes and allergenic potential of foodstuff to develop the next generation of convenience foods (Barba *et al.*, 2015).

HPP Principles

There are three fundamental operational principles underlying HPP, viz; Le-Chatelier's principle, isostatic principle and principle of microscopic ordering.

Le Chatelier's Principle

If a stress is applied on a system in equilibrium, then the system will try to counteract that applied stress and restore the equilibrium, reactions that result in reduced volume will be promoted under high pressure, such reactions may result in inactivation of microorganisms or enzymes (Farkas and Hoover, 2000).

Isostatic Principle (Pascal's Law)

HPP is mass/ time independent; therefore, pressure is transmitted instantaneously and uniformly throughout a sample, and pressure gradients do not exist, so that the size and geometry of the product is irrelevant (Olsson, 1995).

Principle of Microscopic Ordering

At a constant temperature, increase in pressure increases the degree of ordering of molecules. Therefore, pressure and temperature exert antagonistic forces and molecular structure and chemical reactions (Balny and Masson, 1993).

Components and Working of HPP

Two types of pressure generation system which are used in the commercial equipment of the high pressure processing i.e. Direct and indirect compression system. In direct compression system, a pressure vessel is provided with the piston arrangement. In case of indirect compression systems, the fluid is pressurized somewhere else i.e. in pressure medium tank and then this pressurized fluid is loaded in the pressure chamber/vessel of the HPP equipment through or with the help of an intensifier.

The HPP system consist of following components. A high-pressure system consists of a high-pressure vessel and its closure(s), pressure-generation system, temperature control device and material-handling system (Mertens, 1995). The pressure vessel is the most important component of high hydrostatic-pressure equipment. Pressure-transmitting fluids are used in the vessel to transmit pressure uniformly and instantaneously to the products sample. Most widely used fluids are water, glycol solutions, silicone oil, sodium benzoate solutions, ethanol solutions, inert gases and castor oil (Yaldagard *et al.,* 2008). The food products should be packaged in a flexible packaging. The packages are loaded into the high pressure chamber. The vessel is sealed and the vessel filled with pressure transmitting agent. The high pressure is usually carried out with water as a hydraulic fluid to facilitate the operation and compatibility with food materials (Earnshaw, 1996).

Packaging Requirements for HPP

In HPP the food product is generally treated in its primary package form resulting a 'secure unit' until the consumer opens it for the consumption. The packaging material must be able to accommodate up to 15% reduction in volume and return to it is original volume without the loss of barrier properties after decompression (Airtight flexible packages required). The packaging material those are impermeable to oxygen and opaque to light should be used to retain the fresh colour and flavour. To improve the barrier properties of the polymeric films, they are occasionally coated with extremely thin layers (a few nanometers thick) of inorganic compounds such as aluminum oxide and silicon oxide, or metalized by the deposition (approximately 0.01 mm thick) of a thin layer of aluminum (Tao *et al.,* 2014).

Microbial Destruction by HPP

Microbial destruction is the main goal of food processing; beneficial effects of HPP in food are evident only when applied pressures exceed 400 MPa. HPP inactivates most of spoilage and pathogenic bacteria present in milk.

Yeasts, moulds and vegetative bacteria are inactivated by pressures between 300 and 600 MPa. Gram-negative bacteria are inactivated at a lower pressure than Gram-positive bacteria. Spores are more resistant than vegetative cells because of calcium rich dipicolinic acid which protects them from excessive ionization (Smelt, 1998).The level of microbial inactivation depends on the pressure applied, duration of treatment, temperature, environment and initial load and types of microorganisms (Voigt *et al.,* 2015).

In order to kill spores using high pressure, the process is divided in two steps: 1st at lower pressures (50 to 300 MPa) germination process, 2nd at higher pressures (> 400 MPa) that inactivates the germinated spores obtained at the end of the first step (Aouadhia *et al.,* 2012). Non enveloped viruses are usually more pressure resistant than enveloped viruses. It is always advisable to a combination of pressure and temperature to inactivate spores particularly in low acid food.

Impact on Physico-Chemical Properties of Milk Constituents

White colour of milk is due to scattering of light particles by fat globules and casein micelles. Hunter Luminance value (L-value) of milk, generally read as a measure of whiteness (Harate *et al.,* 2003), was reported to reduce by HPP treatment, due to disintegration of casein micelles, thus leading to decreases in the turbidity of milk.

Water

Water content of the food gets compressed by about 4 % at 100 MPa and 15% at 600 MPa. Depression in freezing point of water was also observed at high pressure to -4°C, -8°C, -22°C at 50, 100 and 210 MPa, respectively (Kalichevsky *et al.,* 1995). HPP technique enables sub-zero temperature dairy processing without ice crystal formation. It also facilitates rapid thawing of conventional frozen food.

Proteins

At high pressure disrupts casein micelles, which increase with pressure increment (Huppertz *et al.,* 2006). Caseins show dissociated from the micelle in the following order β-casein>κ-casein > αs1-casein > αs2-casein. At higher pressure treatment (250–300 MPa for >15 minutes) can give significant increases in micelle size and changes in turbidity and lightness of skimmed milk. Viscosity is increased by about 20 %. (Needs *et al.,* 2000). β-lactoglobulin denaturation 90 % at pressures (≥400 MPa) and α-lactalbumin 70% at 800 MPa (Huppertz *et al.,* 2004). Bovine serum albumin showed no denaturation in HPP treated milk (at 100–400 MPa) (Lopez-Fandino *et al.,* 1996). Immunoglobulin show stability to HPP; about 90% of immunoglobulin G (IgG) in colostrum remained in native state after HPP treatment (500 MPa for five minutes) (Indyk *et al.,* 2008).

Fat

Treatment at 100–600 MPa at <40°C does not affect milk and cream fat globule size in milk (Ye *et al.,* 2004). The treatment of cream at 800 MPa for 10 minutes increased fat globule size in cream (Kanno *et al.,* 1998). Treatment at 100–250 MPa may promote the cold agglutination of milk fat globules, which may lead to clusters of fat globules during cold storage leading to faster creaming. At >400 MPa, reduced cold agglutination, and hence reduced creaming rate (Voigt *et al.,* 2015).Critical threshold pressure between 300 and 500 MPa of oxidation in lipids (Medina-Meza *et al.,* 2014).

Minerals

Mineral balance of milk gets affected at high pressure and effect is on both the distribution between colloidal and soluble phase and ionization (Johnston *et al.,* 1992). The increase in the content of soluble calcium by HPP. Solubilization of CCP increases with increasing pressure up to about 400 MPa. The concentration of ionic calcium in milk has been observed to slightly increase, immediately after HP treatment (Lopez-Fandino *et al.,* 1998).

Enzymes

Lipoprotein lipase, xanthine oxidase and lactoperoxidase showed resistant up to pressures up to 400 MPa (Naik *et al.,* 2013). Alkaline phosphatase in milk are partially inactivated at pressures exceeding 600 MPa and are completely inactivated at pressures of 800 MPa (Sakharam *et al.,* 2011). Proteolysis was increased during the storage for low pressure treatment, whereas after 500 MPa, the proteolysis during storage of milk was less than that observed in raw milk. The combination of HP treatment (300–600 MPa, 40–60°C) and homogenization resulted in inactivation of protease activity in milk, which extended its shelf life (Sainz *et al.,* 2009).

Applications in Dairy Industry

Fluid Milk Processing

HP treatment of milk at 680 MPa for 10 min at room temperature to reduction of microorganisms of 5–6 log cycle (Hite, 1899). HP treatment (400 MPa for 15 min or 500 MPa for 3 min) of thermally pasteurized milk increased shelf life by 10 days (Rademacher and Kessler, 1997). The combination of HPP with a bacteriocin (lacticin), synergistic effect in controlling microbial flora of HPP milk without significantly influencing other cheese-making properties (Morgan *et al.,* 2000). Milk treated at 400 MPa results in no significant loss of vitamins like B1 and B6 (Sierra *et al.,* 2000).

Narisawa *et al.* (2008) investigated the effects of skimmed milk and its protein fractions (casein, whey, globulin and albumin) on the injury and inactivation of *Escherichia coli K-12* by HHP. The protective effect of skimmed milk on HHP-mediated inactivation and injury of *E. coli* increased with increases in the skimmed milk concentration.

Cheese

HPP caused casein micelle disruption, whey protein denaturation, increase in milk pH and cheese yield, and reduction in RCT, which indicates its significant potential in the cheese-manufacturing (San Martín-Gonzalez *et al.,* 2006). The HP treatment of milk reduces RCT and 15% increase cheese yield and reduced 30% whey proteins loss in cheese production, probably due to whey proteins and casein interaction (Huppertz *et al.,* 2005).

In cheese manufactured from HP treated milk (at 300 or 400 MPa for 10 minutes), increased β-casein hydrolysis and free amino acids (FAAs) level. Similar results were reported for HP treated Cheddar cheese at 50 MPa for 72 h (Wick *et al.,* 2004). HP-treated (500 MPa) goat milk had higher pH and salt content, showed faster maturation, and strong flavours generation (Trujillo *et al.,* 1999). HPT (500 MPa, 10 min) significantly reduced the level of Listeria monocytogenes in the raw milk and so allowed the production of safer non-thermally processed camembert-type soft cheese (Rastogi, 2013). Evert-Arriagada *et al.,* (2014) studied the effect of pressure 500 MPa (5 min, 16 °C) on starter-free fresh cheeses during cold storage of 21 days. The results showed that pressurized cheeses presented a shelf-life of about 19–21 days when stored at 4°C, whereas control cheese became unsuitable for consumption on 7–8 days.

Ice-cream

HP treatment of whey protein concentrate at 300 MPa for 15 min enhanced the foaming properties, and when added to low-fat ice cream to improved body and texture of ice-cream, increased overrun and foam stability and hardness of ice cream than ice cream added with untreated whey protein (Lim *et al.,* 2008). HP treatment of ice cream mix at 500 MPa for 1 second showed increase in the mix viscosity which help for manufacturing of low-fat and stabilizer-free ice creams with better mouthfeel (Huppertz *et al.,* 2011).

Yogurt

Yogurt made from HP treated milk was less susceptible to undesirable syneresis on storage, due to changes in gel structure and water-binding capacity of milk proteins (Capellas *et al.,* 2003). An extended shelf- life 'Probiotic yogurt' has been developed using pressure treatment of 350–650 MPa at 10–15°C. Yogurt maintained desirable sensory characteristics longer than controls during storage for 4 weeks at refrigerated (4°C) or room (20°C) temperature (Carroll *et al.,* 2004). The application of the high pressure in preliminary treatment of milk used for yoghurt production improved firmness of the curd and low syneresis (Liepa *et al.,* 2016).

Fruit yogurt Prepared by HPT (550 MPa) and stored for 4 weeks at refrigerated (4°C) or room (20°C) temperature. They found that pressure treatment prevented the post acidification of the product and the number of bacteria in the HP-treated yogurt stored at 4°C was maintained at less than the therapeutic minimum level of 106 CFU/ml. They also saw that no microbial spoilage took place in HP-processed sample even after 60 days of storage at 4.4 and 25°C. Moreover, the count of LAB decreased to <10 CFU/ml (Dhineshkumar *et al.,* 2016).

Cream and Butter

When cream was treated at pressure of 600 MPa for up to 2 min, its whipping properties improved and reduced serum loss possibly due to better crystallization of milk fat (Eberhard *et al.,* 1999). HP processing of butter and cream lead to rise in the temperature (8–9°C/100 MPa) (Rasanayagam *et al.,* 2003). HP treatment of pasteurized cream at 450 MPa at 25°C did not alter the fat globules size distribution, pH and its flow behavior (Dumay *et al.,* 1996).

Other Dairy Products

Treatment of colostrum with HP has been shown better retention of biological activity than of heat treatment under certain conditions and ensuring a reasonable shelf life of product (Indyk *et al.,* 2008). The Fonterra Company of New Zealand has patented processes for colostrum preservation using HP treatment (Voigt *et al.,* 2015).

There is a great scope for utilizing HPP for the development of probiotic dairy foods with higher viable count.HPP is also used for preparation of channa and paneer (Sahu, 2010). HP treatment of human milk indicated that with at 400MPa for 5 minutes, helped retaining of all immunoglobulin A (IgA) in milk serum that is susceptible to thermal damage during pasteurization using heat treatment (Permanyer *et al.,* 2010). Acid-set gels made from milk treated at high pressure (600 MPa) for 15 min has improved mechanical properties like gel rigidity and gel breaking strength.

Advantages of HPP

- High pressure is not dependent of size and shape of the food.
- HPP retains food quality, maintains natural freshness, and extends microbiological shelf life.
- HPP results in foods with better taste, appearance, texture and nutrition.
- It can be applied at room temperature thus reducing the amount of thermal energy needed for food products during conventional processing.
- High pressure processing is isostatic (uniform throughout the food); the food is preserved evenly throughout, without any particles escaping the treatment.
- The process is environment friendly since, it requires only electric energy and there are no waste products.
- Clean technology, flexible system for number of products and operation.
- Reduced requirement of chemical additives, and Increased bioavailability (Huang *et al.*, 2017).

Disadvantages of HPP

- High capital and installation cost of equipment (Ginsau, 2015).
- Bacterial spores are very resistant to pressure and require very high pressure for their inactivation. May not inactivate spores so, additional heat treatment is required.
- The residual enzyme activity and dissolved oxygen results in enzymatic and oxidative degradation of certain food components.
- Most of the pressure-processed products need low temperature storage and distribution to retain their sensory and nutritional qualities.

HPP Regulations

The USDA has approved HPP as a non-thermal pasteurization technology that can be used to replace traditional thermal pasteurization in the food industry. The Food and Drug Administration (FDA) in 2009 has approved HPP for production of low acid foods and many food processing industries in USA. The European Community (EC) recently founded a major multinational research project on HPP to make a real assessment of the potential of high pressure technology for commercialization (Huang *et al.*, 2017).

New Trends

HPP is the best option to preserve the functional property of thermosetting bioactive components present in colostrum such as immunoglobulin, lactoferrin and growth factor. High-quality organic food raw materials, fresh local foods with short food miles, and functional health foods are new trends in the field of HPP. HPP technology also can be combined with existing trends in the food sector to boost the development of the food industry. For example, high-quality organic food raw materials, fresh local foods with short food miles, and functional health foods are future development trends in the field of HPP (Huang *et al.*, 2017).

Present status and Indian scenario India is relatively new to the field of high pressure processing. Recently Defence Food Research Laboratory (DFRL), Mysore under the aegis of Defence Research Development Organization (DRDO) has successfully installed the first high pressure processing system in India having a processing capacity of 2 litres and a maximum operating pressure of 900 MPa (Ferstl, 2013).

Recent instances of commercialization of HPP in dairy industry can include HP treated Yogurt and Cheese spread. New opportunities in HPP may include exploring HP induced changes in milk giving functional ingredients, preservation of colostrum and human milk by HPP treatment

Issues & Challenges in HPP of Dairy and Food Industries

Heat transfer under high-pressure and process inhomogeneity. The isostatic rule is also not well accepted, because the change in density at the geometric centre of food may experience different pressure. The determination of properties of milk and milk products under high pressure is a complex task and practically no data exists in this regard. HPP is more costly (up to 20 times) than traditional heat technology. The other important issue is the compression heating of the food materials. All compressible substances change temperature during physical compression, and this is an unavoidable thermodynamic effect.

Conclusions

The HPP is a 'novel' and non-thermal technology has the potential for use as an alternative to thermal processing. However, it cannot be denied that the dairy industry has been comparatively slow to adopt HP processing, as compared to meat, sea-food and juice industry. The major effects of HPP in milk due to dissociation of caseins micelles from colloidal to soluble phase, resulting in reduced turbidity of milk, decreased RCT. Principal hindrances to adoption is the high cost of equipment and low throughput of HPP equipment. Recent instances of commercialization of HPP in dairy industry include HP treated Yogurt and Cheese spread. New opportunities in HPP include exploring HP induced changes in milk giving functional ingredients, preservation of colostrum and human milk by HPP treatment, which may be of interest to the entrepreneurs.

References

Aouadhia, C., Simonin, H., Prévostc, H., de Lamballerie, M., Maaroufi, A. & Mejri, S. (2012). Optimization of pressure-induced germination of Bacillus sporothermodurans spores in water and milk. *Food Microbiology*. 30: 1-7.

Balny, C. & Masson, P. (1993). Effects of high pressure on proteins. *Food Rev. Int.,* 9(4): 611-628.

Barba F. J., Terefe, N. S., Buckow, R., Knorr, D. & Orlien, V. (2015). New opportunities and perspectives of high pressure treatment to improve health and safety attributes of foods. A review. *Food Res. Int.*, 77: 725–742.

Capellas, M., & Needs, E. (2003) Physical properties of yoghurt prepared from pressure-treated concentrated or fortified milks. *Milchwissenschaft,* Vol. 58, pp46–48.

Carroll, T., Ping, C., Harnett, M., & Harnett, J. (2004) Pressure treating food to reduce spoilage. International Patent Wo 2004/032655.

Dhineshkumar, V., Ramasamy, D. & Siddharth, M. (2016). High pressure processing technology in dairy processing: A review. *Asian J. Dairy Food Res.,* 35(2): 87-95.

Dumay, E., Lambert, C., Funtenberger, S. & Cheftel, J. C. (1996). Effect of high pressure on the physiocochemical characteristics of dairy creams and model oilywater emulsion. *Lebensmittel Wissenschaft and Technologie*, 29(7): 606-625.

Earnshaw, R. (1996). High pressure food processing. *Nutrition & Food Science*, 96(2), 8-11.

Eberhard, P., Strahm, W. & Eyer, H. (1999) High pressure treatment of whipped cream, *Agrarforschung*, Vol. 6, pp352-354.

Evert-Arriagada, K., Hernandez-Herrero, M. M., Guamis, B., & Trujillo, A. J. (2014). Commercial application of high-pressure processing for increasing starter-free fresh cheese shelf-life. *LWT-Food Science and Technology*, 55(2), 498-505.

Farkas, D. & Hoover, D. (2000). High Pressure Processing. In: Kinetics of microbial inactivation for alternative food processing technologies. *J. Food Sci. Suppl.,* 65:47-64.

Ferstl, C. (2013). High pressure processing insights on technology and regulatory requirements. Food for Thought Topical Insights. *The National Food Lab White Paper Series* Vol. 10. pp2-6.

Garcia-Risco, M. R., Cortes, E., Carrascosa, A. V. & Lopez-Fandino, R. (1998). Microbiological and chemical changes in high-pressure-treated milk during refrigerated storage. *Journal of Food Protection*, Vol. 61, pp735–737.

Ginsau, M.A. 2015. High pressure processing: A novel food preservation technique. *J. Environ. Sci., Toxicol.Food Technol.*, 9(5): 109-113.

Harate, F., Luedecke, L., Swanson, B. & Barbosa-Canvas, G. V. (2003). Low fat set yoghurt made from milk subjected to combinations of high pressure and thermal processing, *J. Dairy Sci.*, 86: 1074-1082.

Hite, B. H. (1899). The effect of high pressure preservation of milk. Bulletin of the West Virginia Agricultural Experimental Station, 58, pp15–35.

Horie, Y., Kimura, K., Ida, M., Yosida, Y. & Ohki, K. (1991). Jam preservation by pressure pasteurization. *Nippon Nogeiku Kaichi*, 65: 975-980.

Huang, H. W., Wu, S. J., Lu, J. K., Shyu, Y. T. & Wang, C. Y. (2017). Current status and future trends of high-pressure processing in food industry. *Food Contro*, l72: 1-8.

Huppertz, T., Fox, P. F., De Kruif, K. G. & Kelly, A. L. (2006). High pressure-induced changes in bovine milk proteins: a review. Biochimica et Biophysica Acta – Proteins and Proteomics, Vol. 1764: 593–598.

Huppertz, T., Fox, P. F. & Kelly, A. L. (2004). High pressure treatment of bovine milk: effects on casein micelles and whey proteins. *Journal of Dairy Research*, Vol. 71, pp97–106.

Huppertz, T., Hinz, K., Zobrist, M. R., & Fox, P. F. (2005). Effects of high pressure treatment on the rennet coagulation and cheese-making properties of heated milk, *Innovative Food Science and Emerging Technologies*, Vol. 6, Issue 3, pp279-285.

Huppertz, T., Smiddy, M. A., Kelly, A. L. & Goff, H. D. (2011). Effect of high pressure treatment of mix on ice cream manufacture. International Dairy Journal, Vol. 21, pp718–727.

Indyk, H. E., Williams, J. W. & Patel, H. A. (2008). Analysis of denaturation of bovine IgG by heat and high pressure using an optical biosensor. *International Dairy Journal,* Vol. 18, pp359–366.

Johnston, D. E., Austin, B. A. & Murphy, P. M. (1992). Effect of high hydrostatic pressure on milk. *Milchwissenschaft*, 47: 760-763.

Kalichevesky, M. T., Knorr, D. & Lillford, P. J. (1995). Potential applications of high pressure effects on ice water transition. *Trends Food Sci. Technol*., 6: 253-259.

Kanno, C., Uchimura, T., Hagiwara, T., Ametani, M., & Azuma, N. (1998). Effect of hydrostatic pressure on the physicochemical properties of bovine milk fat globules and the milk fat globule membrane, High Pressure Food Science, BioScience and chemistry, The Royal Society of Chemistry.

Liepa, M., Zagorska, J. & Galoburda, R. (2016). High-pressure processing as novel technology in dairy industry: a review. *Research for Rural Development*, Vol. 1, pp76-83.

Lim, S. Y., Swanson, B. G., & Clark, S. (2008). High hydrostatic pressure modifications of whey protein concentrate for improved functional properties. *Journal of Dairy Science*, Vol. 91, pp1299– 1307.

Lopez-Fandino, R., Carrascosa, A. V. & Olano, A. (1996). The effect of high pressure on whey protein denaturation and cheese making properties of raw milk. *J. Dairy Sci.*, 79(6): 923-936.

Medina-Meza, I., Barnaba, G. C. & Barbosa-Canovas, G. V. (2014). Effects of high pressure processing on lipid oxidation: A review. *Innovative Food Science and Emerging Technologies,* Vol. 22, pp1-10.

Mertens, B. (1995). In: New Methods of Food Preservation (G.W. Gould, Ed.), Blackie Academic and Professional, New York, p. 135.

Morgan, S. M., Ross, R. P., Beresford, T., & Hill, C. (2000). Combination of high hydrostatic pressure and lacticin 3147 causes increased killing of Staphylococcus and Listeria. *Journal of Applied Microbiolology*, Vol. 88, pp414–420.

Muntean, M. V., Marian, O., Barbieru, V., Catunescu, G. M., Ranta, O., Drocas, I. & Terhes, S. (2016). High pressure processing in food industry – Characteristics and applications. *Agric. Agril. Sci. Procedia.,* 10: 377–383.

Naik, L., Sharma, R., Rajput, Y. S. & Manju, G. (2013). Application of High Pressure ProcessingTechnology for Dairy Food Preservation-Future Perspective: A Review. *Journal of Animal Production Advances*, Vol. 3, Issue 8, 232-241.

Narisawa, N., Furukawa, S., Kawarai, T., Ohishi, K., Kanda, S., Kimijima, K., Negishi, S., Ogihara, H., and Yamasaki, M. 2008. Effect of skimmed milk and its fractions on the inactivation of Escherichia coli K12 by high hydrostatic pressure treatment. *Int. J. Food Microbiol*, 124: 103–107.

Needs, E. C., Capells, M., Bland, P., Manoj, P., MacDougal, D. B. & Gopal, P. (2000). Comparison of heat and pressure treatment of skimmed milk, fortified with whey protein concentrate for set yoghurt preparation: effects on milk proteins and gel structure. *Journal of Dairy Research*, Vol. 67, pp329-348.

Olsson, S. (1995). Production equipment for commercial use, In: High Pressure Processing of Foods (D. A. Ledward, Johnston DE, Earnshaw RG and Hasting APM, Eds), Nottingham University Press, Nottingham. p. 167.

Permanyer, M., Castellote, C., Ramírez-Santana, C., Audí, C., Perez-Cano, F. J., Castell, M., López- Sabater, M. C., & Franch, A. (2010). Maintenance of breast milk immunoglobulin A after high pressure processing. *Journal of Dairy Science*, Vol. 93, pp877–883.

Rademacher, B. & Kessler, H. G. (1997). High pressure inactivation of microorganisms and enzymes in milk and milk products, High Pressure Research in the Biosciences and Biotechnology, Leuven University Press.

Rao, P. S., Chakraborty, S., Kaushik, N., Kaur, B. P. & Hulle, N. R. S. (2014). High Hydrostatic Pressure Processing of Food Materials, Introduction to Advanced Food Process Engineering, CRC Press.

Rasanayagam, V., Balasubramaniam, V. M., Ting, E., Sizer, C. E., Bush, C. & Anderson, C. (2003) Compression heating of selected fatty food materials during high-pressure processing. *Journal of Food Science*, Vol. 68, pp254–259.

Rastogi, N. K. (2013). High-pressure processing of dairy products. In "Recent Developments in High Pressure Processing of Foods". Springer Briefs in Food, Health, and Nutrition (R.W. Hartel and J.P. Clark Eds.) PP 51-64.

Sahu, J. K. (2010). Coagulation kinetics of high pressure treated acidified milk gel for preparation chhana (an Indian soft cottage cheese). *Int. J. Food Prop.*, 13:1054–1065.

Sainz, C. B., Younce, F. L., Rasco, B., & Clark, S. (2009) Protease stability in bovine milk under combined thermal-high hydrostatic pressure treatment. *Innovative Food Science and Emerging Technologies*, Vol. 10, pp314–320.

Sakharam, P., Prajapati, J. P. & Jana, A. H. (2011). High Hydrostatic Pressure Treatment for Dairy Applications. National seminar `Indian Dairy Industry - Opportunities And Challenges`, 2014. 176-180.

San Martín-Gonzalez, M. F., Welti-Chanes, J. & Barbosa-Cánovas, G. V. (2006). Cheese Manufacture assisted by high pressure. *Food Reviews International*, Vol. 22, pp275–289.

Sierra, I., Vidal, V. C. & Lopez, F. R. (2000)0 Effect of high pressure on the vitamin B1 and B6 content of milk. *Milchwissenschaft*, Vol. 55, No. 7, pp365- 367.

Smelt, J. P. P. M. (1998). Recent advances in the microbiology of high pressure processing. *Trends in Food Science and Technology*, Vol. 9, pp152–158.

Tao, Y., Sun, D. W., Hogan, E. & Kelly, A. L. (2014). High pressure processing of foods: An overview. In "Emerging Technologies for Food Processing" (D.-W. Sun Ed.), Second Edition. Academic Press (an imprint of Elsevier), 32 Jamestown Road, London NW1 7BY, UK. PP 3-24.

Trujillo, A. J., Royo, B., Guamis, B. & Ferragut, V. (1999) Influence of pressurization on goat milk and cheese composition and yield. *Milchwissenschaft*, Vol. 54, pp197–199.

Wick, C., Nienaber, U., Anggraeni, O., Shellhammer, T. H., & Courtney, P. D. (2004). Texture proteolysis and viable lactic acid bacteria in commercial Cheddar cheeses treated with high pressure. Journal of Dairy Research, Vol. 71, 107–115.

Yaldagard M., Seyed A. M. & Tabatabaie F. (2008). African Journal of Biotechnology, 7(16), 2739-2767.

Ye, A., Anema, S. G., & Singh, H. (2004). High-pressure–induced interactions between milk fat globule membrane proteins and skim milk proteins in whole milk. Journal of Dairy Science, Vol. 87, pp4013–4022.

3

Pulsed Electric Fields (PEF) Technology Principle and Application in Food Processing

Himanshu Kumar Singh, Sunil Sakhala, Chandni Dularia and Shamim Hossain

Dairy Technology Division, ICAR-National Dairy Research Institute Karnal, India

Abstract

The demand for safe and high-quality food items has led to the development of numerous unique food processing processes during the past few decades. Consumers today have high standards for the product's sensory quality, functionality, and nutritional worth. They also place a high value on the utilisation of environmentally sustainable food producing methods. Pulsed electric field (PEF) processing is an emerging method of food processing and preservation that uses short bursts of electricity for microbial inactivation (cell-lysis) and causes minimal or no detrimental effect on food quality attributes. PEF can be used mainly for processing liquid and semi-liquid food products. The creation of high electric field intensities, the design of chambers that treat food uniformly while increasing temperature minimally, and the design of electrodes that reduce the effect of electrolysis are some crucial elements of PEF technology. The high field intensities are made possible by storing a significant quantity of energy from a DC power source in a capacitor bank (a collection of capacitors), which is subsequently released in the form of high voltage pulses. This chapter's objective is to provide an overview of PEF's uses in food technology, food processing, food preservation and in the creation of functional foods.

Introduction

Electricity is one of the fundamental phenomena of nature. Electricity or electric current is caused due to the movement of charged particles *i.e.*, electrons. Due to the potential difference between two points in a conductor, electron movement takes place. The potential difference between two points is caused due to the difference in charge density. Electron tends to flow from lower potential to higher potential which causes electricity to flow. In general, the electrons flow from cathode (negative) to anode (positive) but in a wire electricity, electrons flow from anode to cathode when connected to a battery or any electricity source. This is because electricity is considered to be the flow of positive charge which is not so because only electron moves from one point to another in a conductor. So, opposite to the direction of moving electron, flow of positive charge is imagined that drifts from anode (+ve) to cathode (-ve). Batteries are used as source of electricity which consists of two terminals namely, anode (positive potential) and cathode (negative potential).

Electrons are the currency of charge having a net negative charge. Presence of an extra electron in any atom or molecule gives negative charge to that atom while absence of an electron gives positive charge and this is how positive and negative ions are created in the nature. Electricity is said to be the greatest discovery of all time and with this a window of opportunity was opened. Many machines and instruments based on electricity were invented and have transformed the world we are witnessing today. Utilization of electricity has transformed many fields of science and technology and also in the field of food science. Charge starts to build up or organize on the surface of the uncharged object when a charge-bearing object is placed near to it, keeping in mind that they do not touch each other. This building up of charge is due to induction. This can also take place when an object is kept in an active electric field. In the electric field, there is polarity and due to that, induction charging takes place on an object. The object kept in the electric field gets induced charged sides, opposite to the polarity of the electric field.

Non-thermal processes

Non-thermal processes are the methods in which preservation is not primarily due to thermal effects but some other phenomena. There is a slight rise in temperature but that is insignificant concerning food preservation or processing. Potential non-thermal food processing technologies are enlisted below:

a) Pulsed electric field technology

b) High-pressure processing

c) Preservation using UV light

d) Preservation by ionising radiation (irradiation)

e) High-intensity pulsed light technology

f) Application of oscillating magnetic field

Among enlisted non-thermal technologies above, our discussion will be focused on pulsed electric field (PEF) technology.

Working Principle of PEF

High intensity PEF technology treatment (Figure 3.1) is the application of high intensity pulsated electric field on food material placed between two electrodes. As there will be an active electric field between electrodes and exposure of this electric field to microorganisms causes immense changes in the cell membrane permeability. This immense change in the cell membrane is known as **Electroporation.** Electroporation is the generation of pores on the cell membrane which makes it permeable to small molecules, water and other cell constituents. Eventually the cell membrane swells up and ruptures as represented in Figure 3.2. These pores are reversible or irreversible depending on the type of microorganism. The causes of the electroporation are not well understood but induced charges, on the cell membrane surface due to an active high-intensity electric field between electrodes might be a reason. These induced charges change the transmembrane potential of cell membrane *i.e.*, 1 volt larger than the natural transmembrane potential of cell membrane. This is called dielectric rupture theory (Tsong, 1989). The intensity of the electric field is 20 kV or more and the DC (direct current) is used to generate this high-intensity electric field using a series of charged capacitors. DC power is used for charging capacitors and then discharging that energy in the form of high voltage pulses into the processing chamber containing food (Figure 3.1). It is said to be pulsated because electric field in processing chamber is applied in the form of different wave functions of time be it exponential or square. It means that, if PEF is applied exponentially then the voltage will change with time exponentially for each pulse.

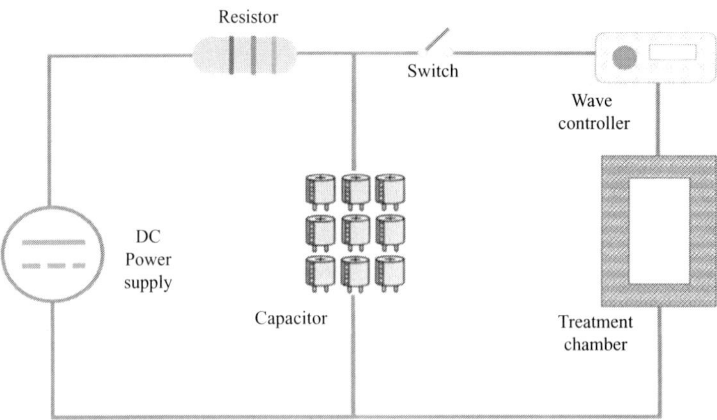

Fig. 3.1: Schematic diagram representing equipment for high-intensity PEF generation

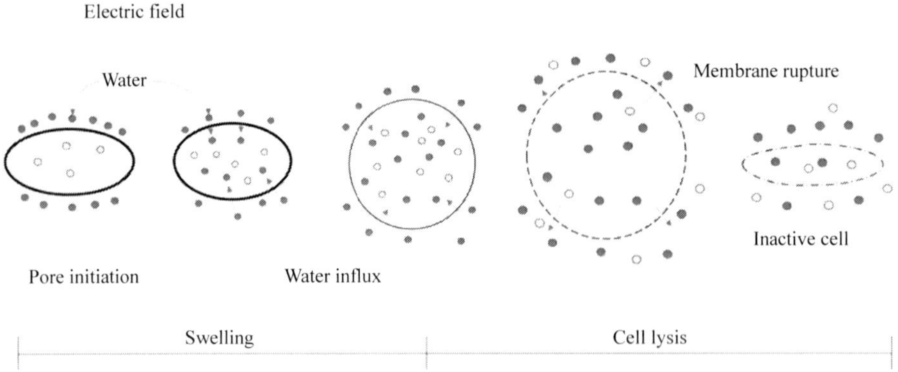

Fig. 3.2: Electroporation and cell inactivation

The concept of PEF is simple, electrical energy with low power is stored in capacitors and then discharge instantaneously with high power levels to the treatment chamber (Vega-Mercado *et al.,* 2007). Components of PEF unit are: DC power supply, charging resistor, discharge switch, capacitors, wave controller, treatment chamber.

PEF in Food Processing

Pasteurization of foods like juices, milk, yoghurt, soups, *etc.* has been effectively accomplished with the help of PEF technology. Food products with poor electrical conductivity and no air bubbles are the only kind of products that can be processed using PEF. To ensure proper treatment, the maximum particle size of liquid must be less than the gap of the treatment region in the chamber. Continuous PEF technology are suitable for liquid products due to their flowable property and therefore they can't be used for solid food products. PEF is also used to improve sugar and other cellular content extraction from plant cells, such as sugar beet cells. It is also useful in lowering the sludge volume in wastewater. Orange, apple, and cranberry juice are just a few examples of the fruit juices with low viscosity and electrical conductivity that have successfully undergone PEF processing. More than a 3-10g reduction in orange juice (Qin et al., 1998) and apple juice was noted in recent research (Evrendilek *et al.,* 2000).

Moreover, according to a recent study of PEF-treated orange juice stored at 4°C for 112 days, there was less browning than thermally pasteurised juice, which was explained by the conversion of ascorbic acid to furfural. The colour change in fruit juices (subject to prolonged storage) was also reportedly less in juices treated by PEF (Yeom *et al.,* 2000).

PEF treatment is successful on liquid items including milk, fruit juices, liquid eggs and any other pumpable food products, substantial study has been conducted to put the procedure into practice on an industrial scale. Besides achieving microbiological safety of food products, some of the key reasons of interest include flavour freshness, economic viability, improvements in functional and textural features, and longer shelf life (Dunn, 2019). Apple juice, orange juice, milk, liquid eggs, and brine solutions are the liquid items to which PEF technology has been most commonly applied (Qin *et al.,* 1996).

There are particular uses for each non-thermal technology in terms of the kinds of foods that can be processed. PEF is one of the most promising non-thermal processing technique for microbial inactivation, and they have the potential to replace pasteurisation of liquid foods. PEF has the ability to pasteurise a variety of foods by exposing them to high voltage brief pulses kept at temperatures below 30–40°C, similar to pasteurisation but without the thermal component. PEF technology's fundamental definition is based on the utilisation of high-intensity pulsed electric fields (l0-80 kV/cm) for disrupting cell membranes. Induced electric fields perforate microbial membranes using electroporation, a biotechnology technique that facilitates bacterial DNA exchange. When membrane potentials are induced, they frequently cause cell damage and death if they surpass a certain value.

Application of PEF in Food Processing

A method of pasteurising milk using a low-frequency alternating electric field was created at the start of the 1990s. In 1960, a German engineer named Doevenspeck received a patent for a technique that involved high-voltage electric waves and assisted in dismantling the cell structure of food items (Toepfl *et al.*, 2006). The effectiveness of PEF technology in food processing is heavily influenced by processing variables such as pulse shape, pulse breadth, electric field strength, treatment time, pulse frequency, polarity, temperature, and treatment in batch or continuous flow systems. Optimization of PEF parameters is needed for each specific application of PEF. Some examples are presented in Table 3.1.

Table 3.1: Examples of process conditions and effects of using PEF in food processing

Material	PEF parameters	Effect of PEF	References
Drying			
Basil (*Ocimum basilicum L.*) leaves	65 pulses of 650 V/cm, 150 ls pulse width, 760 ls between pulses	Drying time reduced 57% for air drying, 33% for vacuum drying and 25% for freeze drying	Telfser & Galindo, 2019
Potato tissue	300–400 V/cm	Decreased drying temperature approx. 20 degrees	Lebovka *et al.*, 2007
Extraction			
Citrus fruits and peel	3 kV/cm—fruits 10 kV/cm—peel	Increased yield of juice by 25% for oranges, 37% for pomelos and 59% for lemon, improved extraction of polyphenols to 50%	El Kantar *et al.*, 2018
Blueberry fruits (*Vaccinium myrtillus L.*)	1,3 and 5 kV/cm, 10 kJ/kg	Increasing the juice yield (+28%) compared to the untreated sample. The juice obtained had higher total phenolic content (+43%), total anthocyanin content (+60%) and antioxidant activity (+31%)	Bobinaite *et al.*, 2015
Freezing			

Material	PEF parameters	Effect of PEF	References
Baby spinach leaves	Two trains of bipolar, rectangular pulses with amplitude of 350 V, with 10s interval between trains. Each train consisted of 500 pulses of 200 ls pulse width and 1600 ls of space between the pulses (frequency 500 Hz)	Freezing tolerance is improved by applying vacuum impregnation and PEF in the presence of cryoprotectants	Demir *et al.*, 2018
Beef muscle	1,4 kV/cm, 20 ls, 50 Hz, 250 kJ/ kg (combined with freezing and thawing)	Microstructural changes in meat tissue, improved tenderness and purge loss	Faridnia *et al.*, 2015
Preservation			
Milk	25.7 kV/cm for 34 ls after heating to 55 C and maintained for 24 s and heat treatment at 63 C for 30 min or at 73 C for 15 min	Inactivation of alkaline phosphatase. Reduced xanthine (30%) and plasmin oxidase (7%) activity	Sharma *et al.*, 2017
Fresh berries	2 kV/cm, pulse width 1 ls and 100 pulses per second for 2, 4 and 6 min + disinfectant solution (60 ppm peracetic acid [PAA])	The reduction of *E. coli* and *Listeria innocua* without changing the colour and appearance of blueberries The softening of the berry structure Conc. of anthocyanins and phenolic compounds increased by 10 and 25%, respectively	Jin *et al.*, 2017

Drying

The sample's resistance to diffusion is decreased after being pre-treated with PEF to break down the cell structure, the mass and heat transfer rates between the cells and their surroundings are increased (Barba *et al.*, 2015). Alam *et al.* (2018) conducted research on the effects of initial PEF treatment on drying kinetics, changes in colour, and texture in sliced parsnip and carrot. Compared to the untreated samples, the drying time was cut by 28% at 70°C and 21% at 60°C. According to Wiktor *et al.* (2016), the effective water diffusion coefficient of the PEF-treated carrot samples increased by 16.7 %, drying time was lowered by 8.2 %, and the samples' lightness and redness were higher than they were in the undamaged tissue. Ostermeier *et al.* (2018), looked into how drying onions affected by a PEF pre-treatment. According to the study, a rise in cell disintegration produced by an increasing electric field strength—up to 1.07 kV/cm—facilitated the escape of moisture to the product's surface. For PEF pre-treated onion sample dried at 45°C, the greater diffusion resulted in a 30% reduction in drying time. Telfser & Galindo (2019) investigated the impact of reversible permeabilization as a pre-treatment basil (*Ocimum basilicum* L.) leaf before air drying at 40°C, vacuum drying, and freeze drying. When PEF was used, drying times for air drying, vacuum drying, and freeze drying were all reduced by 57%, 33% and 25%, respectively. According to a sensory panel, PEF-treated and vacuum-dried samples were the ones that resembled fresh leaves in terms of colour and scent. The use of PEF also hastens the drying of other foods, such as paprika, apples, coconuts, potatoes, and carrots (Ade-Omowaye *et al.,* 2001).

Freezing

One significant drawback of freezing food is that the ice crystals that develop can damage the tissue, causing the items (such as soft fruits and leafy vegetables) to lose their shape and become soggy after thawing. Customers do not accept them in this form. It has been shown that infant spinach leaves can be made more resistant to freezing by using PEF. In the presence of cryoprotectants such trehalose, sucrose, glucose, and fructose, PEF was applied via vacuum impregnation. After the cycle of freezing and thawing, the combination of these techniques ensured that the leaf cells were still viable and the leaves preserved their turgor (Demir *et al.,* 2018). After being submerged in various cryoprotectant and texturizing agents, carrot discs treated with PEF had higher firmness than the control sample after thawing (Shayanfar *et al.,* 2014). In another study done on potato strips demonstrated that PEF treatment alone (without texturizing and antifreeze chemicals) was an ineffective pre-treatment technique, but when combined with $CaCl_2$ and trehalose, potato strips preserved structural integrity, firmness, and colour after thawing (Shayanfar *et al.,* 2013). It's interesting to note that using PEF along with vacuum infusion, cryoprotectants, frozen and thawed strawberries did not improve their texture. However, this procedure improved the thawed fruits' ability to retain their colour (Velickova *et al.,* 2018). The use of PEF technology along with freezing or freeze-drying changes the time and rate of freezing. For instance, the study by Jalte *et al.* (2009) demonstrated that PEF pre-treatment can shorten the freezing period, speed up the freeze-drying process, and enhance the freeze-dried potato's quality. Similar to this, Wiktor *et al.* (2015) found that the effect of PEF on the total freezing time and total thawing time of apple tissue were decreased by 3.5-17.2 percent and 71.5 percent, respectively. The authors concluded that electroporation of multicellular tissues led to better connections between intra- and extracellular content allowing increased probability of ice nucleation and faster ice propagation after freezing and correspondingly shortening the freezing time.

Food Preservation

Many things, including the growth of microorganisms and the action of endogenous enzymes, can lead to food deterioration. In contrast to the conventional pasteurisation approach, the PEF technology reduces the loss of the original taste, colour, texture, nutrients, and other thermolabile components present in food while also partially inactivating pathogenic germs and enzymes (Syed *et al.,* 2017). This makes it a promising addition to or replacement for conventional thermal pasteurisation. For liquid items with low viscosity and electrical conductivity, such as milk and juices, PEF can be utilised successfully.

Microbial Inactivation

To make milk and dairy products safe for human consumption, they are treated thermally using a variety of techniques. Inadequate pasteurisation of milk results in product deterioration and the growth of harmful bacteria such *Escherichia coli*, *Listeria* species, and *Pseudomonas*. Nutrient losses occur during the high-temperature treatment (Ercolini *et al.,* 2009). In addition to inactivating microorganisms at low temperatures, PEF have negligible effects on the food product's nutritional and sensory qualities. Gram-negative and Gram-positive bacteria in whole milk that has already reached 50°C are rendered inactive by PEF (Sharma *et al.,* 2014). When kept at 4°C, thermally preserved milk can remain microbiologically stable for 21 days. However, heat has negative consequences that include denaturing of whey proteins, lactose, non-enzymatic browning, and impairment to the creaming capabilities. In order to boost the efficiency of bacterial inactivation and extend the period of consumption, PEF technology can be employed in conjunction with heat, antimicrobial chemicals, membrane filtration, and UV radiation. Sharma *et al.* (2017) suggested in their study that the milk samples treated with PEF under the following conditions: 25.7 kV/cm for 34 ls after heating to 55°C and maintaining it for 24 s; heat treatment at 63°C/30 min; or at 73°C/15 min. Alkaline phosphatase inactivation was similar across all samples. After 21 days of refrigerator storage, the PEF-treated sample's reduced xanthine (30%) and plasmin oxidase (7%) activity were comparable to those of the milk sample that had not been processed at all. All milk samples underwent storage with increased lipolytic activity and decreased pH. According to Hemar *et al.* (2011), when milk is treated with high field strengths, PEF can have an impact on viscosity and particle size but has no effect on whey proteins or milk pH. Jin *et al.* (2017) investigated the effects of PEF on blueberries that have been artificially grafted with *Listeria innocua* and *E. coli* populations. *E. coli* and *Listeria innocua* were reduced as a result of PEF and PAA (60 ppm peracetic acid), however the colour and appearance of blueberries were unaffected. The softening of the berry structure was the only drawback to the process. The concentrations of phenolic compounds and anthocyanins both rose by 10% and 25%, respectively. To lower *Listeria innocua* in a milk-based smoothie, Palgan *et al.* (2012) coupled PEF and Mano Thermos Sonication (MTS). The research demonstrated that the most efficient method for inactivating *L. innocua* which resulted in a mean reduction of 5.6 log cfu/ml was the administration of MTS followed by PEF.

Spore Inactivation

Endospores appear to be unaffected by PEF processing, despite the fact that some papers claim that spore inactivation can be achieved under particular severe conditions. Compared to vegetative cells, spores exhibit greater resistance to PEF because of their tiny size, limited permeability, dehydration, and mineralization. Therefore, pasteurisation (not sterilisation) can currently be accomplished only with PEF treatment. However, successful inactivation of endospores can be achieved by combining the administration of PEF with other techniques, such as thermal treatment. For example, Siemer *et al.* (2014) observed a 3-log cycle inactivation of *B. subtilis* spores under the following process conditions: an electric field strength of 9 kV/cm, an inlet temperature of 80°C, and the addition of 10% sugar to the medium.

Enzyme Inactivation

More strong PEF treatments are needed to inactivate enzymes since they are less susceptible to PEF's effects than bacteria are, but the exact mechanism underlying this occurrence is still unclear. PEF is thought to have both electrochemical and thermal effects, which alter the structure and conformation of enzymes and induce their deactivation (Terefe *et al.*, 2013). PEF did not significantly change the physicochemical and sensory properties of grape juice, which is sensitive to the action of several enzymes, but it did lessen the activity of polyphenol oxidase and peroxidase. The relative activity of a few enzymes was significantly influenced by the length, intensity, and frequency of PEF action; this effect was eliminated as the aforementioned parameters increased (Marselles-Fontanet & Martin-Belloso, 2007).

Extraction of Bioactive Compounds

One of the most popular methods in the industry for obtaining valuable compounds is extraction, which often entails subjecting a sample to chemical and/or heat treatment. According to numerous studies, applying a PEF during the extraction process can increase its effectiveness, shorten the extraction process, and minimise any damage to the retrieved nutrients. PEF has been applied to enhance intracellular chemical extraction from fruits and vegetables. According to Luengo *et al.* (2013), PEF treatment improved the quantity of polyphenols that could be extracted from tomatoes and grapes. The extraction of polyphenols from the leaves of borage (*Borago officinalis L.*) and their antioxidant activity were both improved by the use of this approach. The increase in pulse intensity was proportional to the quantity of polyphenols extracted and to their antioxidant capabilities, and it also decreased the extraction time (Segovia *et al.*, 2014). Soliva-Fortuny *et al.* (2017) investigated the impact of PEF on the concentration of phenols, flavonoids, and flavan-3-ol as well as on the antioxidant capacity of apples which were held at two temperatures (4 and 22°C) for 48 hours. The apple treated with the mildest electric field conditions showed the greatest increase in total phenol content (13%) and flavone-3-ol (92%). In comparison to the untreated samples, apples that had undergone PEF also had 43% more antioxidant activity. The impact of PEF on the extraction of water-soluble phenolic components from onions as well as the antioxidant activity of the extracts were both studied by Liu *et al.* (2018). The results showed that after PEF treatment and water extraction, the yield of water-soluble phenolic and flavonoid chemicals extracted from onion significantly increased by 2.2 and 2.7 times, respectively, in comparison to control. The antioxidant activity of extracts was found to increase with both treatment time and electric field intensity, according to the authors. El Kantar *et al.* (2018) looked into how PEF affected citrus fruits (orange, pomelo and lemon). A pulsed electric field was used to treat fruits and peel at field voltages of 3 kV/cm and 10 kV/cm, respectively. PEF processing boosted the extraction of polyphenols to 50% and raised the output of juice by 25% for oranges, 37% for pomelos, and 59% for lemons.

Starch Modification

Modification of potato, corn, wheat, and cassava starches is possible using PEF (Han *et al.*, 2009; Hong *et al.*, 2018; Hong *et al.*, 2016). Along with the increase in field strength (1.25–5 kV/cm and 30–50 kV/cm), the researchers found the rearrangement and destruction of starch molecules as well as a decrease in the gelatinization characteristics, viscosity, and crystallinity. When PEF was applied, the amount of fast digested starch increased in potato, wheat, and pea starches (PEF intensities of 2.86, 4.29, 5.71, 7.14, and 8.57 kV/cm, 600 Hz of pulse frequency, and 6 ls of pulse width) as well as waxy rice starch (30, 40, and 50 kV/cm) (Zeng *et al.,* 2016). According to Hong *et al.* (2018), PEF treatment can significantly improve starch modification techniques like acetylation (PEF parameters: pulse frequency of 1000 Hz; field intensity of 1.25, 2.50, 3.75, and 5.00 kV/cm; pulse duration time of 40 ls). Utilizing PEF to assist starch modification techniques can improve process effectiveness, speed up reaction times, and conserve reagents.

Conclusion

The selected current and future uses of PEF in the food sector were covered in this chapter. The desire for food produced using environmentally friendly practises and the growing interest of customers in goods that resemble fresh foods and have excellent nutritional values are two factors that are driving the development of innovative technology in food processing. PEF is a technique that makes use of high voltage and high amplitude electric waves. The product is placed between the electrodes in the chamber and is given brief electrical impulses (from microseconds to milliseconds each) of high voltage (typically 10-80 kV/cm). By lowering the temperature and length of the extraction process, this technology can produce products in a way that is both more energy-efficient and environmentally beneficial. PEF can be used for pasteurisation, the improvement of processes like drying, freezing, or extraction, but it can also promote the development of functional foods that include, for example, readily absorbed ions of elements necessary for human body function. Worldwide research is being done on PEF technologies. Although this technology has undergone substantial research and commercial PEF systems are already operational in some nations, the majority of the results still apply to laboratory-scale operations.

References

Ade-Omowaye, B. I. O., Angersbach, A., Taiwo, K. A., & Knorr, D. (2001). Use of pulsed electric field pre-treatment to improve dehydration characteristics of plant based foods. *Trends in Food Science & Technology*, *12*(8), 285-295.

Alam, M. R., Lyng, J. G., Frontuto, D., Marra, F., & Cinquanta, L. (2018). Effect of pulsed electric field pretreatment on drying kinetics, color, and texture of parsnip and carrot. *Journal of food Science*, *83*(8), 2159-2166.

Barba, F. J., Parniakov, O., Pereira, S. A., Wiktor, A., Grimi, N., Boussetta, N., ... & Vorobiev, 3E. (2015). Current applications and new opportunities for the use of pulsed electric fields in food science and industry. *Food Research International*, *77*, 773-798.

Bobinaite, R., Pataro, G., Lamanauskas, N., Satkauskas, S., Viskelis, P., & Ferrari, G. (2015). Application of pulsed electric field in the production of juice and extraction of bioactive compounds from blueberry fruits and their by-products. *Journal of food science and technology*, *52*(9), 5898-5905.

Demir, E., Dymek, K., & Galindo, F. G. (2018). Technology allowing baby spinach leaves to acquire freezing tolerance. *Food and Bioprocess Technology*, *11*(4), 809-817.

Dunn, J. (2019). Pulsed electric field processing: an overview. Pulsed electric fields in food processing, 1-30.

El Kantar, S., Boussetta, N., Lebovka, N., Foucart, F., Rajha, H. N., Maroun, R. G., & Vorobiev, E. (2018). Pulsed electric field treatment of citrus fruits: Improvement of juice and polyphenols extraction. *Innovative Food Science & Emerging Technologies*, *46*, 153-161.

Ercolini, D., Russo, F., Ferrocino, I., & Villani, F. (2009). Molecular identification of mesophilic and psychrotrophic bacteria from raw cow's milk. *Food microbiology*, *26*(2), 228-231.

Evrendilek, G. A., Jin, Z. T., Ruhlman, K. T., Qiu, X., Zhang, Q. H., & Richter, E. R. (2000). Microbial safety and shelf-life of apple juice and cider processed by bench and pilot scale PEF systems. *Innovative Food Science & Emerging Technologies*, *1*(1), 77-86.

Faridnia, F., Ma, Q. L., Bremer, P. J., Burritt, D. J., Hamid, N., & Oey, I. (2015). Effect of freezing as pre-treatment prior to pulsed electric field processing on quality traits of beef muscles. *Innovative Food Science & Emerging Technologies*, *29*, 31-40.

Han, Z., Zeng, X. A., Zhang, B. S., & Yu, S. J. (2009). Effects of pulsed electric fields (PEF) treatment on the properties of corn starch. *Journal of Food Engineering*, *93*(3), 318-323.

Hemar, Y., Augustin, M. A., Cheng, L. J., Sanguansri, P., Swiergon, P., & Wan, J. (2011). The effect of pulsed electric field processing on particle size and viscosity of milk and milk concentrates. *Milchwissenschaft-Milk Science International*, *66*(2), 126.

Hong, J., Zeng, X. A., Buckow, R., Han, Z., & Wang, M. S. (2016). Nanostructure, morphology and functionality of cassava starch after pulsed electric fields assisted acetylation. *Food Hydrocolloids*, *54*, 139-150.

Hong, J., Zeng, X. A., Han, Z., & Brennan, C. S. (2018). Effect of pulsed electric fields treatment on the nanostructure of esterified potato starch and their potential glycemic digestibility. *Innovative Food Science & Emerging Technologies*, *45*, 438-446.

Jalte, M., Lanoisellé, J. L., Lebovka, N. I., & Vorobiev, E. (2009). Freezing of potato tissue pre-treated by pulsed electric fields. *LWT-Food Science and Technology*, *42*(2), 576-580.

Jin, T. Z., Yu, Y., & Gurtler, J. B. (2017). Effects of pulsed electric field processing on microbial survival, quality change and nutritional characteristics of blueberries. *LWT*, *77*, 517-524.

Lebovka, N. I., Shynkaryk, N. V., & Vorobiev, E. (2007). Pulsed electric field enhanced drying of potato tissue. *Journal of Food Engineering*, *78*(2), 606-613.

Liu, Z. W., Zeng, X. A., & Ngadi, M. (2018). Enhanced extraction of phenolic compounds from onion by pulsed electric field (PEF). *Journal of Food Processing and Preservation*, *42*(9), e13755.

Luengo, E., Álvarez, I., & Raso, J. (2013). Improving the pressing extraction of polyphenols of orange peel by pulsed electric fields. *Innovative Food Science & Emerging Technologies*, *17*, 79-84.

Marsellés-Fontanet, Á. R., & Martin-Belloso, O. (2007). Optimization and validation of PEF processing conditions to inactivate oxidative enzymes of grape juice. *Journal of food engineering*, *83*(3), 452-462.

Ostermeier, R., Giersemehl, P., Siemer, C., Töpfl, S., & Jäger, H. (2018). Influence of pulsed electric field (PEF) pre-treatment on the convective drying kinetics of onions. *Journal of Food Engineering*, *237*, 110-117.

Palgan, I., Muñoz, A., Noci, F., Whyte, P., Morgan, D. J., Cronin, D. A., & Lyng, J. G. (2012). Effectiveness of combined pulsed electric field (PEF) and manothermosonication (MTS) for the control of Listeria innocua in a smoothie type beverage. *Food Control*, *25*(2), 621-625.

Qin, B. L., Barbosa-Canovas, G. V., Swanson, B. G., Pedrow, P. D., & Olsen, R. G. (1998). Inactivating microorganisms using a pulsed electric field continuous treatment system. *IEEE Transactions on Industry Applications*, *34*(1), 43-50.

Qin, B. L., Pothakamury, U. R., Barbosa□Cánovas, G. V., Swanson, B. G., & Peleg, M. (1996). Nonthermal pasteurization of liquid foods using high□intensity pulsed electric fields. *Critical Reviews in Food Science & Nutrition*, *36*(6), 603-627.

Segovia, F. J., Luengo, E., Corral-Pérez, J. J., Raso, J., & Almajano, M. P. (2015). Improvements in the aqueous extraction of polyphenols from borage (Borago officinalis L.) leaves by pulsed electric fields: Pulsed electric fields (PEF) applications. *Industrial Crops and Products*, 65, 390-396.

Sharma, A. K., Sharma, C., Mullick, S. C., & Kandpal, T. C. (2017). Potential of solar industrial process heating in dairy industry in India and consequent carbon mitigation. *Journal of Cleaner Production*, *140*, 714-724.

Sharma, P., Bremer, P., Oey, I., & Everett, D. W. (2014). Bacterial inactivation in whole milk using pulsed electric field processing. *International Dairy Journal*, *35*(1), 49-56.

Shayanfar, S., Chauhan, O. P., Toepfl, S., & Heinz, V. (2013). The interaction of pulsed electric fields and texturizing□antifreezing agents in quality retention of defrosted potato strips. *International Journal of food Science & Technology*, *48*(6), 1289-1295.

Shayanfar, S., Chauhan, O. P., Toepfl, S., & Heinz, V. (2014). Pulsed electric field treatment prior to freezing carrot discs significantly maintains their initial quality parameters after thawing. *International Journal of Food science & Technology*, *49*(4), 1224-1230.

Siemer, C., Toepfl, S., & Heinz, V. (2014). Inactivation of Bacillus subtilis spores by pulsed electric fields (PEF) in combination with thermal energy II. Modeling thermal inactivation of B. subtilis spores during PEF processing in combination with thermal energy. *Food Control*, *39*, 244-250.

Soliva-Fortuny, R., Vendrell-Pacheco, M., Martín-Belloso, O., & Elez-Martínez, P. (2017). Effect of pulsed electric fields on the antioxidant potential of apples stored at different temperatures. *Postharvest Biology and Technology*, *132*, 195-201.

Syed, Q. A., Ishaq, A., Rahman, U. U., Aslam, S., & Shukat, R. (2017). Pulsed electric field technology in food preservation: a review. *Journal of Nutritional Health & Food Engineering*, *6*(6), 168-172.

Telfser, A., & Galindo, F. G. (2019). Effect of reversible permeabilization in combination with different drying methods on the structure and sensorial quality of dried basil (*Ocimum basilicum* L.) leaves. *Lwt*, *99*, 148-155.

Terefe, N. S., Kleintschek, T., Gamage, T., Fanning, K. J., Netzel, G., Versteeg, C., & Netzel, M. (2013). Comparative effects of thermal and high pressure processing on phenolic phytochemicals in different strawberry cultivars. *Innovative Food Science & Emerging Technologies*, *19*, 57-65.

Toepfl, S., Heinz, V., & Knorr, D. (2006). Pulsed electric fields (PEF) processing of meat. In *13th World Congress of Food Science & Technology 2006* (pp. 591-591).

Tsong, T. Y. (1989). Electroporation of cell membranes. *Electroporation and electrofusion in cell biology*, 149-163.

Vega-Mercado, H., Gongora-Nieto, M. M., Barbosa-Canovas, G. V., & Swanson, B. G. (2007). Pulsed electric fields in food preservation. In *Handbook of food preservation* (pp. 801-832). CRC Press.

Velickova, E., Tylewicz, U., Dalla Rosa, M., Winkelhausen, E., Kuzmanova, S., & Romani, S. (2018). Effect of pulsed electric field coupled with vacuum infusion on quality parameters of frozen/thawed strawberries. *Journal of Food Engineering, 233*, 57-64.

Wiktor, A., Nowacka, M., Dadan, M., Rybak, K., Lojkowski, W., Chudoba, T., & Witrowa-Rajchert, D. (2016). The effect of pulsed electric field on drying kinetics, color, and microstructure of carrot. *Drying Technology*, *34*(11), 1286-1296.

Wiktor, A., Schulz, M., Voigt, E., Witrowa-Rajchert, D., & Knorr, D. (2015). The effect of pulsed electric field treatment on immersion freezing, thawing and selected properties of apple tissue. *Journal of Food Engineering, 146*, 8-16.

Yeom, H. W., Streaker, C. B., Zhang, Q. H., & Min, D. B. (2000). Effects of pulsed electric fields on the quality of orange juice and comparison with heat pasteurization. *Journal of Agricultural and Food Chemistry*, *48*(10), 4597-4605.

Zeng, F., Gao, Q. Y., Han, Z., Zeng, X. A., & Yu, S. J. (2016). Structural properties and digestibility of pulsed electric field treated waxy rice starch. *Food Chemistry*, *194*, 1313-1319.

4

Cold Plasma Technology in Dairy and Food Industry

Akashkumar K. Solanki, Radhika Govani and Ashwin S. Hariyani

Assistant Professor, College of Dairy Science, Kamdhenu University, Amreli, Gujartat, India

Abstract

Thermal pasteurization and sterilization are predominantly used in the dairy industry due to their efficacy in improving the product safety and shelf life. Thermal processing have negative effect on the overall nutritional quality of dairy and food products. Therefore, modern dairy and food industries are shifting towards non-thermal processing method for retaining the overall nutritional quality of food and dairy products. Hence, food industries are approaching towards green and novel technology which are energy efficient as well as provide superior qulaties of food products. Among different green technology cold plasma (CP) technology is one of the novel techniques which are largely utilized in the current era. Plasma is a state of matter in which a significant number of atom and/or molecules are electrically charged or ionized. This technique not only provides better nutritional property but also provides higher shelf life food by destruction of spoilage causing microorganism by different mechanism. This unique not only provide superior quality food but it also has positive impact on the structural modification of macro and micro molecules of food. Hence, this technique opens a new aspect for designing functionally modified food or food additives for different application. Although, plasma technology has proven its efficacy in food processing sector but few researches proved that plasma processed high fat foods develop off flavor, and undesirable texture and color changes are also observed. Therefore, more researches are require to be carried out to optimize CP parameters for different food applications. Also, it is require to identify and analyse different cost parameters for large scale industrial applications.

Introduction

Thermal heating methods are used from long time to decontaminate the food products from microorganism and therefore increase its shelf life and ultimately make the product safe for human consumption. But these methods diminishthe sensory, physicochemical and nutritional properties of food (Barba *et al.*, 2012). Also, the cost of generation of heat in manufacture of food product make the product costlier in thermal processing and also create environmental issue. So, researchers are moving towards the alternate process i.e. non-thermal process and it may solve the problems associated with thermal processes. Non-thermal methods can be a solution to replace the severe heating process. These methods include High Pressure Processing (HPP), Pulsed Electric Field (PEF), Microfiltration (MF), Ultraviolet light (UV), irradiation, ultrasoundand Cold Plasma (CP) techniques. These methods have minimum detrimental effect on physical, organoleptic and nutritional properties of food, also effective against spoilage causing microorganisms (Kaluwahandi *et al.*, 2020).

Cold plasma is a distinctive, reasonably inexpensive and environment friendly technology. The term plasma is the Greek word (meaning "moldable substances) was first described by the chemist Irving Langmuir in 1928. He described it as a non-thermal technology and it is the fourth state of matter. In CP process reactive oxygen species (ROS) is generated using combination of active gas, electrically energized ions and atoms (free electrons) by applying magnetic, electric or thermal energy (Laroussi, 2015). Cold plasma can be used for microbial inactivation or surface decontamination for food products, such as meat, grains, dairy, fresh vegetables and fruits. Moreover, it can modify surface properties of food and/or packaging materials as well as enhancement of mass transfer on the surface (Kaluwahandi *et al.*, 2020).

There are different methods to generate plasma i.e. Plasma jets, Dielectric Barrier Discharges (DBD), corona discharges, and microwave discharges. In most methods plasma is generated at atmospheric pressure (Surowsky *et al.*, 2015).

Plasma is a very hot ionised gas which is made up of equal numbers of positively charged particles (protons) and negatively charged particles (electrons) (Ekezie *et al.*, 2017). When some external energy is applied to the atoms the high energy causes the electrons to strip away from the atomic nuclei and produces various reactive plasma products such as electrons, ions, neutrons, protons and reactive oxygen, atomic oxygen (O), ozone (O3), hydroxyl radicals (OH+) and nitrogen species (N2, NO, NO2, nitric oxide radical NO+). The external energy sources can be electrical energy, magnetic current, radiofrequency waves, intense ultraviolet or laser light. The energy produced is depending upon the type of gas used and amount of energy applied (frequency/watt) used for generation of ROS (Phan *et al.,* 2017).

Based on the method of generation, pressure and the relative temperature, plasma can be classified in to two different groups they are 1) Non-thermal plasma 2) Thermal plasma. Thermal plasma contains contain gas species and electrons having same temperature of around 10000°K under high pressure are thermodynamically equilibrium in nature. Hence, Thermal plasma has found its use in effectively treating the hazardous metal wastes (Pankaj *et al.,* 2018). Non-thermal plasma are also called as cold plasma or non-equilibrium plasma is partially ionised gas which are produced under atmospheric/vacuum temperature of about 30-60°C (Thirumdas *et al.,* 2015). Cold plasma contains various gaseous species possess same energy of above moderate room temperature but the electron poses higher temperature of 20,000K with higher energy. Fast growing demand for fresh produce poses the food industries to supply minimally processed food in a safe manner to the consumer. As a result, cold plasma technique can be a promising technique for preserving food by destroying microorganisms without affecting its quality (Misra *et al.,* 2011; Mishra *et al.,* 2016).

Principle and Mechanism of Decontamination

Plasma sterilization effect was first documented and patented in the year 1968 by Menashi. When the food surface contaminants are exposed to reactive species produced by plasma there will be an accumulation of electrostatic forces at place where the high energy flows. The energy flows further induce radical bombardment action and hence cell lysis occurs. The impact of radical bombardment causes the lesions on the surface makes the microbial cell impotent to repair quickly which results in cell destruction. This phenomenon is termed as "plasma etching".Plasma etching causes DNA and chemical bonds denaturation, thus produces an antimicrobial effect on the cell (Menashi, 1968).

Factors Affecting Plasma Decontamination

- Power level to generate the plasma
- Gaseous mixture and Intensity of gases species
- Length of exposure
- Flow rate, Pressure and design of the system
- Milleu factors - Relative humidity, pH and nature of sample (Ekezie *et al.,* 2017; Cullen *et al.,* 2018)

Action of Cold Plasma on Bacterial Cell

Methods of Generation of Cold Plasma

Plasma target chamber consist of simple gas such as air or nitrogen or the system with mixture of noble gases such as helium, argon and neon to attain plasma state. Ionised gas will be generated with the application of electric field or any external energy. For atmospheric cold plasma generation DBD method, atmospheric plasma jet discharge, corona discharge and gliding arc discharge are commonly used as it requires mild conditions for processing operation (Niemira, 2012; Mehmood *et al.,* 2018).

Dielectric Barrier Discharge

This method uses two flat metal electrodes which are covered with dielectric material. Neutral gas or any noble gaseous mixture moves between two electrodes in a closed target chamber and is ionized to generate plasma products. One electrode is connected to high voltage circuit and the other is grounded. The power consumption ranges between 10 and 100 W is used for its operation (Shimizu *et al.,* 2018).

Jet discharge

Plasma jet devices are made up of two concentric electrodes. The outer electrode is grounded and the inner electrode is connected to external energy source such as radio frequency source and creates RF (Radiofrequency) energy. Thus interacts with the working gas in the target chamber causes ionization and exits through nozzle and gives 'jet-like' appearance (Zhang, 2015).

Gliding Arc Discharge

Gliding arc discharge follows periodic phenomenon that produces an auto-oscillating plasma species between two electrodes submerged in a laminar or turbulent flow. Plasma discharge starts from narrow end (termed as equilibrium stage), where the connecting electrodes of opposite polarity are joined together and it grows between lengths of the interelectrode. The non-equilibrium phase starts when the arc exceeds its critical value. Plasma column undergoes heat loss when begins to exceeds the energy supplied by the power source. At that point, plasma rapidly cools and produces cold plasma (Khalili *et al.,* 2018).

Corona Discharge Plasma

In this process, plasma is produced by non-uniform electric field strength under atmospheric pressure. Corona discharge appears near sharp points and along thin wires and it is represented in below figure. In highly non-uniform electric field, gases exceeds its breakdown strength and produces weakly ionised plasma with some luminosity. Corona discharges are best suited for food sterilization applications (Antao, 2009).

Exposure Methods

There also different exposure methods studied by Cullen *et al.,* (2018) to deliver the plasma species to the defined target (Sarangapani *et al.,* 2018).

A. Direct exposure

B. Indirect or remote exposure

C. Plasma-activated water

A. Direct Exposure

This method involves the direct exposure of plasma discharge onto the food surface by jet plasma or DBD method. It maximises the food interaction with the short-lived reactive gas species, UV (Ultraviolet rays) and electrons. However this method is not suitable for the sensitive food products which are complex in nature (Sarangapani *et al.,* 2018; Okazaki *et al.,* 2014).

B. Indirect or Remote Exposure

In this approach, food products are placed in the target chamber which are some distance away from the plasma discharge. This method is suitable for sensitive food products which are fragile or contain susceptible tissues. By this method, one can achieve the uniform plasma discharge over certain produce (Sarangapani *et al.,* 2018; Misra *et al.,* 2014).

C. Plasma Activated Water

In this technique water is activated for a period of time with several metastable species of cold plasma which results in the activation of relatively long-lived reactive species such as hydrogen peroxide, nitrates, and nitrites in the water. The resulted plasma water is then used for treatment of certain fresh produce by immersion, spraying or frozen as an active ice (Sarangapani *et al.,* 2018; Wu *et al.,* 2018).

Food Applications of Cold Plasma Treatment

Cold plasma technology shows promising dimensions for various sectors of food processing. It includes:

Dairy Processing Sector

Cold Plasma technology has tested on various milk products include Whole milk, skim milk, UHT (Ultra High Temperature) milk and sliced cheese and concluded that it could become an alternative milk processing technique. It is less likely affected the colour, pH, flavour and nutritional value of the milk products. It also inactivated contaminating microorganisms and alkaline phosphatase enzyme in few seconds (Song *et al.,* 2009; Coutinho *et al.,* 2018). DBD plasma for sterilisation of milk at the voltage of 3kV for 3min at 500Hz frequency, results showed that plasma is a very effective for killing the bacteria completely present in raw milk (Aslan, 2016). In case of sliced cheese more than 8 log reduction were observed (Song *et al.,* 2009). So, cold plasma technology could probably be an effective technique in enhancing their shelf life and keeping quality.

Food Packaging

CP treatments are utilised for the food packaging and biofilms treatments to enhance its antimicrobial and mechanical properties. Also, make positive impact on the various packaging properties include glazing, sealability, moisture/gas barrier property etc. It is considered to be reliable and cost effective technology (Rajvanshi, 2008; Niemira, 2012). To avoid the post packaging contamination and can be used for industrial scale manufacturing (Misra *et al.,* 2014). On RTE (Ready to Eat) meat inside PE (Polyethylene) bags were studied and stated that plasma reduced the counts of Listeria innocua (Rød *et al.,* 2012).

Grain Science and Processing Sector

Food grains and legumes were investigated for *Aspergillus spp.* and *Penicillum spp.* before and after treatment with plasma products showed significant log reduction after exposure for 15min (Selcuk *et al.,* 2008). Depending upon the method of generation, treatment time and type of starch present in the food grains, cold plasma species are able to alter the starch properties. Cold plasma reactive species acts on food grains and causes surface modification, molecular degradation/granular etching or corrosion. Application of cold plasma was effectively studied on various food grain starches such as banana starch, Rice starch, zein, pea protein isolates, Brown rice and Basmati rice to improve its functional properties by surface and molecular modification of starch (Ezeh *et al.,* 2018). CP helps in improving the swelling capacity, decreasing the cooking temperature, pasting viscosity, water solubility and water holding capability of food grains. When oxygen containing cold plasma are used for food rich in fats it may induce lipid oxidation and reduce the acceptability (Gavahian *et al.,* 2018). Plasma when treated on banana starch at different voltages (30kV,

40kV, 50kV) for 3min time interval, it does not show any changes in the level of resistant starch and amylose content but increased the relative crystallinity and gelatinization temperature. Hence it was concluded that plasma could be a righteous tool to modify the characteristics of banana starch and other types of starches (Wu *et al.,* 2018). Non-thermal fluidised bed plasma were used for the decontamination of maize grains, significant log reduction was found and well established (Dasan *et al.,* 2016). Bacterial counts of *Bacillus cereus*, *Bacillus subtilis* and *E. Coli* were tested on brown rice using plasma. High antioxidant activity were observed on brown rice when treated with plasma and that could probably increase the nutritional value of the consumer (Chen *et al.,* 2016).

Meat and Egg Processing Sector

Application was reported on beef, pork and chicken meat quality, microbial decontamination and shelf life extension. The result states that the cold plasma species are effective against *E. coli*, salmonella species, *L. monocytogenes*, yeast and mold species on meat surface (Rod *et al.,* 2012; Misra and Jo, 2017; Lee *et al.,* 2011). Decreases the immobilisation of water in protein myofibrillar network and changes its functional properties of packed meat (Wang *et al.,* 2016). Cold plasma have positive effects on surface decontamination of egg shell membrane against *S. enteritidis* and *S. typhimurium* microorganism (Ragni *et al.,* 2010). Atmospheric plasma jets were checked on the surface of sliced ham and chicken meat. The result showed a significant log reduction of 6.52 when treated with nitrogen and oxygen mixture type (Song *et al.,* 2009).

Fruits and Vegetable Processing Sector (F&V)

Cold plasma treatments on fruits and vegetable products includes berries, cherries, Apple, melon, Kiwi etc. were studied. Results proclaimed that CP treatments on the surface of F &V (Fruits & Vegetables) alters the pH and acidity of the food produce. This changes occurs when active species of plasma reacts with moisture on the surface. It is also found that the treated produce shows slight changes in texture (firmness) and colour during their storage period. Colour loss was observed on kiwi fruit and orange fruit juice (Kovacevic *et al.,* 2016). Fresh and cut produce and blue berries and results demonstrated that CP treatments on F & V was effective against aerobic bacteria (Misra *et al.,* 2014; Lacombe *et al.,* 2015). Similarly works on apple surfaces, melons and mangoes shows that there is a significant reduction in the counts of salmonella and *E. coli* after treating with plasma (Tappi *et al.,* 2014; Tappi *et al.,* 2016). Therefore, microbial decontamination using plasma on fruits and vegetables is found to have a positive result with some negative impacts during its storage period.

Waste Water (Effluent) Treatment

A major issue faced by food industry since water coming out of food industry is with high concentration of organic loads. Various thermal, chemical and filtration techniques are used for waste water treatments. ROS (Reactive Oxygen Species) of cold plasma have been reported to cause prompt changes in the degradation or decomposition of liquid waste. Plasma jet exposure at 25kV for 150sec a were used for treating industrial waste coming out of tomato processing plant and for blackberry & beetroot waste water at the rate of 180 sec exposure showed the significant reduction in bacterial counts. Plasma also reduced E. coli counts and endotoxins compounds in the waste water up to 90.22% (Mohamed *et al.,* 2016; Sarangapani *et al.,* 2016).

Agriculture Sector

Agrochemical residues (like pesticides, insecticides etc.) are identified to cause many human health disorder as they contains potentially toxic elements discharged during cultivation and processing to control crop infestation and weeds (Sarangapani *et al.,* 2016; Bourke *et al.,* 2018; Misra *et al.,* 2014). In package treatment were done for pesticides residues present in water and strawberries with DBD plasma discharge for 5-8min. High dense pesticide compounds were degraded in to smaller chemical compounds possess less toxicity than parental compounds (Sarangapani *et al.,* 2017). Seed germination is enhanced when treated with plasma and found to increase water imbibition capacity of seeds and reduction in the microbial growth (Randeniya and De groot, 2015).

Miscellaneous

Mycotoxins are the undesirable secondary metabolite produced by fungi which are thermally and chemically stable. Jet plasma treatment on walnuts eliminated Aspergillus flavus when it is exposed with plasma products for 10min (Amini and Ghoranneviss, 2016). chemical compound Similarly, CP treatments on almonds, Hazelnuts, Black pepper and Red pepper were studied and stated that it is effective against mycotoxin production and surface contaminating microbes salmonella and Bacillus species (Deng *et al.,*2007; Hertwig *et al.,*2015).

Advantages

- Microbial inactivation efficiency can be achieved at low temperature.
- Suitable for treating sensitive raw and fresh food products.

- Requires less power input for operation.
- Doesn't alter or damage the key food nutrients.
- Reduces the risk caused by thermal and chemicals processing of food materials.
- Reduces water usage and solvent system for processing.
- CP don't alter the sensory and nutritional properties of food materials.
- Plasma is environmentally safe once the reactive species are withdrawn from the power supply.
- Equipment cost is low when least cost noble gases are used for processing.

(Bartos *et al.,* 2017; Dey *et al.,* 2016)

Limitations

- Treatment of bulky and irregularly shaped food is difficult.
- Restricted volume and size of the food for treatment.
- Several ROS species has limited penetration into food products.
- It may affects the sensory and nutritional attributes of the food to some extent during processing.
- It may accelerate lipid oxidation and causes negative impact.

(Mandal *et al.,* 2018; Niemira, 2012)

Conclusion

Currently, plasma systems are not commercially available as a sterilizing tool inthe food industry, mainly because they come in many size, shape, and state, and the area has not attracted the interest of physicists and engineers to a sufficient degree. Medical scientists and physicists have already established a good collaboration, and now some commercial scale results can be observed. Therefore, important aspects of this technology are still immature, particularly concerning its use in food. The application of NTP to food products must be studied in depth to supply a basis for the feasibility of plasma for large-scale commercial production. Once food security concerns are clarified, plasma processing must be scaled up for industrial applications.

References

Amini, M., & Ghoranneviss, M. (2016). Effects of cold plasma treatment on antioxidants activity, phenolic contents and shelf life of fresh and dried walnut (Juglansregia L.) cultivars during storage. *Lwt*, *73*, 178-184.

Antao, D. S. (2009). *A study of Direct Current Corona Discharges in Gases and Liquids for Thin Film Deposition* (Doctoral dissertation, Drexel University).

Aslan, Y. (2016). The Effect of Dielectric Barrier Discharge Plasma Treatment on the Microorganisms Found in Raw Cow's Milk. *Türkiye Tarımsal Araştırmalar Dergisi*, *3*(2), 169-173.

Barba, F. J., Esteve, M. J., & Frigola, A. (2012). High-pressure treatment effect on physicochemical and nutritional properties of fluid foods during storage: a review. *Comprehensive Reviews in Food Science and Food Safety,* 11, 307-322.

Bartos, P., Kriz, P., Havelka, Z., Bohata, A., Olsan, P., Spatenka, P. & Dientsbier, M. (2017). Plasma technology in food industry: mini-review. *Kvasny Prumysl*, *63*(3), 134-138.

Bourke, P., Ziuzina, D., Boehm, D., Cullen, P. J., & Keener, K. (2018). The potential of cold plasma for safe and sustainable food production. *Trends in Biotechnology*, *36*(6), 615-626.

Chen, H. H., Chang, H. C., Chen, Y. K., Hung, C. L., Lin, S. Y., & Chen, Y. S. (2016). An improved process for high nutrition of germinated brown rice production: Low-pressure plasma. *Food Chemistry*, *191*, 120-127.

Coutinho, N. M., Silveira, M. R., Rocha, R. S., Moraes, J., Ferreira, M. V. S., Pimentel, T. C., ... & Cruz, A. G. (2018). Cold plasma processing of milk and dairy products. *Trends in Food Science & Technology*, *74*, 56-68.

Cullen, P. J., Lalor, J., Scally, L., Boehm, D., Milosavljević, V., Bourke, P., & Keener, K. (2018). Translation of plasma technology from the lab to the food industry. *Plasma Processes and Polymers*, *15*(2), 1700085.

Dasan, B. G., Boyaci, I. H., &Mutlu, M. (2016). Inactivation of aflatoxigenic fungi (Aspergillus spp.) on granular food model, maize, in an atmospheric pressure fluidized bed plasma system. *Food Control*, *70*, 1-8.

Deng, S., Ruan, R., Mok, C. K., Huang, G., Lin, X., & Chen, P. (2007). Inactivation of Escherichia coli on almonds using nonthermal plasma. *Journal of Food Science*, *72*(2), M62-M66.

Dey, A., Rasane, P., Choudhury, A., Singh, J., Maisnam, D., &Rasane, P. (2016). Cold plasma processing: A review. *J. Chem. Pharm. Sci*, *9*, 2980-2984.

Ekezie, F. G. C., Sun, D. W., & Cheng, J. H. (2017). A review on recent advances in cold plasma technology for the food industry: Current applications and future trends. *Trends in Food Science & Technology*, *69*, 46-58.

Ezeh, O., Yusoff, M. M., & Niranjan, K. (2018). Nonthermal processing technologies for fabrication of microstructures to enhance food quality and stability. In *Food Microstructure and Its Relationship with Quality and Stability* (pp. 239-274). Woodhead Publishing.

Gavahian, M., Chu, Y. H., Khaneghah, A. M., Barba, F. J., & Misra, N. N. (2018). A critical analysis of the cold plasma induced lipid oxidation in foods. *Trends in Food Science & Technology*, *77*, 32-41.

Hertwig, C., Reineke, K., Ehlbeck, J., Knorr, D., & Schluter, O. (2015). Decontamination of whole black pepper using different cold atmospheric pressure plasma applications. *Food Control*, *55*, 221-229.

Kaluwahandi, N. S., Wei, L., & Muthukumarappan, K. (2020). Opportunities and Challenges of Cold Plasma in Food Processing. In *2020 ASABE Annual International Virtual Meeting* (p. 1). American Society of Agricultural and Biological Engineers.

Khalili, F., Shokri, B., Khani, M. R., Hasani, M., Zandi, F., & Aliahmadi, A. (2018). A study of the effect of gliding arc non-thermal plasma on almonds decontamination. *AIP Advances*, *8*(10), 105024.

Kovacevic, D. B., Putnik, P., Dragovic-Uzelac, V., Pędisic, S., Jambrak, A. R., & Herceg, Z. (2016). Effects of cold atmospheric gas phase plasma on anthocyanins and color in pomegranate juice. *Food Chemistry*, *190*, 317-323.

Lacombe, A., Niemira, B. A., Gurtler, J. B., Fan, X., Sites, J., Boyd, G., & Chen, H. (2015). Atmospheric cold plasma inactivation of aerobic microorganisms on blueberries and effects on quality attributes. *Food Microbiology*, *46*, 479-484.

Laroussi, M. (2015) Low-Temperature Plasma Jet for Biomedical Applications. A Review," in *IEEE Transactions on Plasma Science*: 43(3), 703-712.

Lee, H. J., Jung, H., Choe, W., Ham, J. S., Lee, J. H., & Jo, C. (2011). Inactivation of Listeria monocytogenes on agar and processed meat surfaces by atmospheric pressure plasma jets. *Food Microbiology*, *28*(8), 1468-1471.

Mandal, R., Singh, A., & Singh, A. P. (2018). Recent developments in cold plasma decontamination technology in the food industry. *Trends in Food Science & Technology*, 80, 93-103.

Mehmood F., Kamal T. & Ashraf U. (2018). Generation and Applications of Plasma (An Academic Review).

Menashi W. P. (1968). Treatment of surfaces. US Patent, 3, 383-163.

Mishra, R., Bhatia, S., Pal, R., Visen, A., & Trivedi, H. (2016). Cold plasma: emerging as the new standard in food safety. *Res InvInt J EngSci*, *6*, 15-20.

Misra, N. N., & Jo, C. (2017). Applications of cold plasma technology for microbiological safety in meat industry. *Trends in Food Science & Technology*, *64*, 74-86.

Misra, N. N., Patil, S., Moiseev, T., Bourke, P., Mosnier, J. P., Keener, K. M., & Cullen, P. J. (2014). In-package atmospheric pressure cold plasma treatment of strawberries. *Journal of Food Engineering*, *125*, 131-138.

Misra, N. N., Tiwari, B. K., Raghavarao, K. S. M. S., & Cullen, P. J. (2011). Nonthermal plasma inactivation of food-borne pathogens. *Food Engineering Reviews*, *3*(3-4), 159-170.

Mohamed, A. A. H., Al Shariff, S. M., Ouf, S. A., &Benghanem, M. (2016). Atmospheric pressure plasma jet for bacterial decontamination and property improvement of fruit and vegetable processing wastewater. *Journal of Physics D: Applied Physics*, *49*(19), 195401.

Niemira, B. A. (2012). Cold plasma decontamination of foods. *Annual Review of Food Science and Technology*, *3*, 125-142.

Niemira, B. A. (2012). Cold plasma reduction of Salmonella and Escherichia coli O157: H7 on almonds using ambient pressure gases. *Journal of Food Science*, *77*(3), M171-M175.

Okazaki, Y., Wang, Y., Tanaka, H., Mizuno, M., Nakamura, K., Kajiyama, H., Kano, H., Uchida, H., Kikkawa, F., Hori, M., & Toyokuni, S. (2014). Direct exposure of non-equilibrium atmospheric pressure plasma confers simultaneous oxidative and ultraviolet modifications in biomolecules. *Journal of Clinical Biochemistry and Nutrition*, *55*(3), 207-215.

Pankaj, S. K., Wan, Z., & Keener, K. M. (2018). Effects of cold plasma on food quality: A review. *Foods*, *7*(1), 73-83.

Phan, K. T. K., Phan, H. T., Brennan, C. S., & Phimolsiripol, Y. (2017). Nonthermal plasma for pesticide and microbial elimination on fruits and vegetables: an overview. *International Journal of Food Science & Technology*, *52*(10), 2127-2137.

Ragni, L., Berardinelli, A., Vannini, L., Montanari, C., Sirri, F., Guerzoni, M. E., & Guarnieri, A. (2010). Non-thermal atmospheric gas plasma device for surface decontamination of shell eggs. *Journal of Food Engineering*, *100*(1), 125-132.

Rajvanshi, A. K. (2008). Irving Langmuir. *Resonance*, *13*(7), 619-626.

Randeniya, L. K., & de Groot, G. J. (2015). Non□thermal plasma treatment of agricultural seeds for stimulation of germination, removal of surface contamination and other benefits: A review. *Plasma Processes and Polymers*, *12*(7), 608-623.

Rød, S. K., Hansen, F., Leipold, F., & Knøchel, S. (2012). Cold atmospheric pressure plasma treatment of ready-to-eat meat: Inactivation of Listeria innocua and changes in product quality. *Food Microbiology*, *30*(1), 233-238.

Sarangapani, C., Misra, N. N., Milosavljevic, V., Bourke, P., O'Regan, F., & Cullen, P. J. (2016). Pesticide degradation in water using atmospheric air cold plasma. *Journal of Water Process Engineering*, *9*, 225-232.

Sarangapani, C., O'Toole, G., Cullen, P. J., & Bourke, P. (2017). Atmospheric cold plasma dissipation efficiency of agrochemicals on blueberries. *Innovative Food Science & Emerging Technologies*, *44*, 235-241.

Sarangapani, C., Patange, A., Bourke, P., Keener, K., & Cullen, P. J. (2018). Recent advances in the application of cold plasma technology in foods. *Annual Review of Food Science and Technology*, *9*, 609-629.

Selcuk, M., Oksuz, L., & Basaran, P. (2008). Decontamination of grains and legumes infected with Aspergillus spp. and Penicillum spp. by cold plasma treatment. *Bioresource technology*, *99*(11), 5104-5109.

Shimizu, K., Kristof, J., & Blajan, M. G. (2018). Applications of Dielectric Barrier Discharge Microplasma. In *Atmospheric Pressure Plasma-from Diagnostics to Applications*. IntechOpen.

Song, H. P., Kim, B., Choe, J. H., Jung, S., Moon, S. Y., Choe, W., & Jo, C. (2009). Evaluation of atmospheric pressure plasma to improve the safety of sliced cheese and ham inoculated by 3-strain cocktail *Listeria monocytogenes*. *Food Microbiology*, *26*(4), 432-436.

Surowsky, B., Schlüter, O., & Knorr, D. (2015). Interactions of non-thermal atmospheric pressure plasma with solid and liquid food systems: a review. *Food Engineering Reviews*, *7*(2), 82-108.

Tappi, S., Berardinelli, A., Ragni, L., Dalla Rosa, M., Guarnieri, A., & Rocculi, P. (2014). Atmospheric gas plasma treatment of fresh-cut apples. *Innovative Food Science & Emerging Technologies*, *21*, 114-122.

Tappi, S., Gozzi, G., Vannini, L., Berardinelli, A., Romani, S., Ragni, L., & Rocculi, P. (2016). Cold plasma treatment for fresh-cut melon stabilization. *Innovative Food Science & Emerging Technologies*, *33*, 225-233.

Thirumdas, R., Sarangapani, C., & Annapure, U. S. (2015). Cold plasma: a novel non-thermal technology for food processing. *Food biophysics*, *10*(1), 1-11.

Wang, J., Zhuang, H., Hinton Jr, A., & Zhang, J. (2016). Influence of in-package cold plasma treatment on microbiological shelf life and appearance of fresh chicken breast fillets. *Food Microbiology*, *60*, 142-146.

Wu, T. Y., Sun, N. N., & Chau, C. F. (2018). Application of corona electrical discharge plasma on modifying the physicochemical properties of banana starch indigenous to Taiwan. *Journal of Food and Drug Analysis*, *26*(1), 244-251.

Zhang, S. (2015). Atmospheric pressure RF plasma jet: characterization of flow and O2 chemistry. Eindhoven, Netherlands: Technische Universiteit Eindhoven.

5

Aptamer Next Generation Analytical Tool for Dairy Industry

***Ronit Mandal*[1] *and Payal Karmakar*[2]**

[1]*Faculty of Land and Food Systems, University of British Columbia Vancouver-V61 1Z4, British Columbia Canada*
[2]*Division of Dairy Chemistry, National Dairy Research Institute Karnal-132001, Haryana, India*

Abstract

Due to rapid industrial development and urbanization, the food consumption behavior has changed drastically in the last decades. This has also increased the risk of foodborne illness. With growing concerns on food safety, interventions and strategies are being investigated. The methods of food analyses based on antibodies like ELISA and other immunoassay methods are used to a great extent. In the last decade, the research based on aptamer technology has evolved, which is quicker and less expensive than the former. Aptamers, which are short DNA or RNA sequences, and their derived biosensors are used to detect and quantify several target molecules like bacterial cells, enzymes, toxins, antibiotics and other molecules in food and dairy products. Thus, there has been numerous application of this technology in dairy industry. The main aim of this chapter is to explain the concepts to the readers about the aptamers and their fabrication process (systematic evolution of ligands by exponential enrichment or SELEX). Some recent applications of aptamers in the dairy industry in the field of detection of pathogens, toxins, allergens, adulterants have also been summarized.

Introduction

The last two decades have seen rapid growth and development in the industrial sector as well as urbanization has increased. Due to globalization and mass production of commodities, the situation in the modern world nothing like ever before. Food and dairy industries are also not left out from this massive expansion. Due to changing behavior and food consumption habits too, there has been a surge in the risk of foodborne illness. This has created a problem in terms of public health and sustainability. In United States alone, there are more than 82 million cases of foodborne illness annually (Mandal *et al.,* 2020). Also, the modern consumers are more aware and demand safe and nutritious food.

Food safety issues and foodborne illnesses are manifested by the way of several physical, chemical and biological hazards. These include physical hazards such as dirt and extraneous matters, chemical hazards like heavy metals (like mercury, lead), toxins (aflatoxin, patulin, bacterial toxins), drugs and pesticide residues and biological hazards like microorganisms (salmonella, *Listeria, Escherichia coli*). Use of unregulated additives, poor quality food ingredients and adulteration are also some of the problems that are plaguing the food and dairy industries.

The goal of food safety, regulations and food processing is to minimize the incidences of foodborne illnesses and diseases. Detection of potential hazards is an important measure for ensuring the safety of food products in the domain of quality control and quality assurance in the food industries. Conventional methods or tools of food safety analyses are based on chromatography, such as gas or liquid chromatography combined with mass spectrometry. These methods are highly accurate and sensitive. But these are operated in laboratory settings, thus expensive, time-consuming and require well-trained and patient testing personnel. Some alternatives to the above-mentioned conventional techniques include antibody-based assays or immunoassays. These include enzyme-linked immunosorbent assay (ELISA), western blotting or gold immunochromatographic assay (GICA). These are rapid and cheaper detection techniques and are widely used in the industries. Some important challenges faced while using immunoassays are that difficulty in selection and raising of antibodies for immunogens and toxicants, ethical use of animals and nonspecific binding under real time analyses. This led to the exploration of novel testing and detection methods.

Molecular ligands or chemocentric detection methods have been introduced to offer promising solutions in this regard. The developments in the *in vitro* nucleic acid selection and amplification process has led to the discovery of specific molecular segments from nucleic acids that can bind to a wide spectrum of target molecules with high specificity and affinity. Aptamers are such oligonucleotide ligands or short single-stranded DNA or RNA segments that have the ability to bind target molecules like bacteria, proteins, antibiotics, sugars, toxins etc. (Paniel and Noguer, 2019; Schmitz *et al.,* 2020). The techniques which is used to obtain these aptamers is called systematic evolution of ligands by exponential enrichment (SELEX) process. It was developed by Truek and Gold in 1990 (Dong *et al.*, 2014). The aptamers bind with the targets using molecular interactions like hydrophobic bonds, hydrogen bonds, van der Waal forces etc. to recognize them. Some important applications of aptamers in dairy and food industry are resonance and electrochemical biosensors, usage in slid phase extraction columns, aptamer-nanoparticle colorimetry, dynamic light scattering. The main aim of this book chapter is to elucidate the readers about the salient features of aptamer used in food and dairy industry. Some results of the applications related to the aptamers that are published are also discussed.

Fundamentals

Aptamers–structure and Properties

Aptamers term was derived from the Latin word 'aptus' which means 'to fit'. Thus, the meaning of aptamer is to fit or bind to specific target molecules. Chemically, they are single stranded DNA or RNA molecules or oligonucleotide with 50-100 bases. They vary in sizes ranging from 1-2 nm with 7.5-32 kDa. Overall, it has been observed that the DNA aptamers are more stable than RNA aptamers, however, their binding ability and specificity are same (Schmitz *et al.,* 2020). Typical structure and target binding of aptamer is given in Figure 5.1.

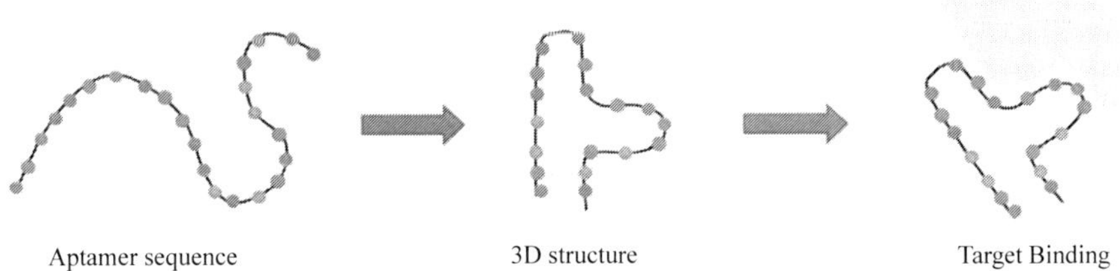

Fig. 5.1: Typical aptamer structure and target binding

The aptamers are unique in nature having random nucleotide sequences, with similar 3' and 5' regions. Aptamers can take shapes or structure of stable three-dimensional configurations in the aqueous phase, for instance triplexes, hairpin, loops, pseudoknots, staples or G-quadruplexes (Liu and Zhang, 2015; Schmitz *et al.,* 2020). The high specificity and binding affinity with target molecules which is characterized by their equilibrium dissociation constant (K_d) which ranges between picomolar (pM) levels and nanomolar (nM). This parameter has special relevance with respect to the applications in therapeutics and fabrication of drug delivery systems. Till now, hundreds of aptamers have been selected out having very high affinity with target molecules like cells, growth factors, transcription factors, proteins, peptides, enzymes, antibiotics, heavy metals, organic compounds and even pathogens. They can be used as enzyme, toxin and hormone inhibitors. Aptamers can be stored at room temperature showing their great stability. Modifications in the structures of aptamers can also enhance their resistance and stability against harsh environmental conditions. For instance, modifying aptamers at their 3' end with thymidine or biotin/biotin-streptavidin, also, adding cholesterol in 5' end can enhance their resistance to nuclease degradation. They can also be combined with nanostructures like gold nanoparticles or carbon nanotubes (Schmitz *et al.,* 2020). By virtue of these affinities they have been used in the biology and medical fields. Thus, they have a great potential too in the filed of food analysis and food safety.

Sensors based on aptamer technology (aptasensors) for detection of target molecules can be classified into optical transduction types (such as fluorescence based or colorimetric based), which give signal in terms of visual appearance and electrochemical signal based aptasensors are which generate measurable electrical signals. Aptamers are advantageous in many respects as compared to the antibody/immunoassay counterparts. The main differences between the aptamers and antibodies have been summarize in Table 5.1.

Table 5.1: Comparison of aptamers and antibodies (*Source*: Dong *et al.*, 2014)

Criteria	Antibodies	Aptamers
Fabrication method	Expensive, time consuming	Less expensive, efficient process
Selection	Under physiological conditions	Under various conditions
Environmental stability	Poor	Fair
Shelf-life	Lower	Prolonged
Detection	Good	Better
Target molecules	Not for toxins and nonimmunogens	Any targets
Binding dissociation constant	nM-pM	nM-pM
Modifications	Limited and difficult	Possible
Target sites	Epitopes determined by immune system	Aptatopes determined by investigator
Cross reactivity	Not attainable	attainable

SELEX Process

The aptamer is selected and screened by systematic evolution of ligands by exponential enrichment process. The SELEX process was first introduced by Tuerk and Gold in 1990, whereby they used a method for selecting RNA aptamers that can bind to T4 DNA polymerase (gp43) (Dong *et al.*, 2014; Schmitz *et al.,* 2020). SELEX is an iterative screening technique whereby a library of random chemically synthesized oligonucleotides is created using *in vitro* combinatorial methods. This consists of about 10^{13}-10^{15} variants which have about 20-80 nucleotides. Each sequence is flanked by different polymerase chase reaction (PCR). These variants assume different shapes and structures. The quality of initial libraries determines success of the SELEX experiments. After the population of library, the library sequences are cultured with the target molecule (at low concentrations) under specified buffer solutions for letting the oligonucleotide-target complex form. The targets can be immobilized on a solid support for easier separation of the unbound molecules (Rothlisberger and Hollenstein, 2018). The complexes formed are washed to screen off weakly-bound ad unbound complexes by rigorous washing. Also, other techniques like magnetic cell sorting, centrifugation, column chromatography, capillary electrophoresis or membrane processing using nitrocellulose filter (Liu and Zhang, 2015; Schmitz *et al.,* 2020). This constituted the first round of selection. The nucleotide-target complexes are eluted at high temperature and urea, EDTA addition. The oligonucleotides amplified by using PCR proliferation method. Then a new nucleic acid (double stranded DNA) pool is generated. The new pool is again screened for aptamers in the next cycle iteratively. This way the initial pool of oligonucleotide library is reduced to obtain potential candidate for aptamers. The number of cycles that are performed depend on the required affinity and specificity. Usually around 20 different cycles are performed. Some parameters that affect the total number of cycles are—method of screening), target properties and concentrations, library type, concentration of aptamer candidates (Dong *et al.,* 2014; Schmitz *et al.,* 2020). Once the rounds of selection are completed, the screened aptamers are cloned into vector and sequenced. Sometimes, the aptamers are subjected to further modifications, whereby additional functional groups, reporter groups, spacers. The affinity and specificity are also tested. The SELEX procedure mentioned above is often time-consuming and difficult. It was also an *in vitro* experiment which pose challenges when translated into real samples. Therefore, several variants of the SELEX process have emerged. Some of these are magnetic bead based SELEX, capillary electrophoresis SELEX, tailored SELEX, whole cell SELEX, FluMag SELEX, genomic SELEX, photo SELEX, subtractive SELEX, crosslinking SELEX, toggle SELEX, etc. Detailed study on SELEX variants are given in the literature (Liu and Zhang, 2015; Darmostuk *et al.*, 2015; Rothlisberger and Hollenstein, 2018). The SELEX process is shown in Figure 5.2.

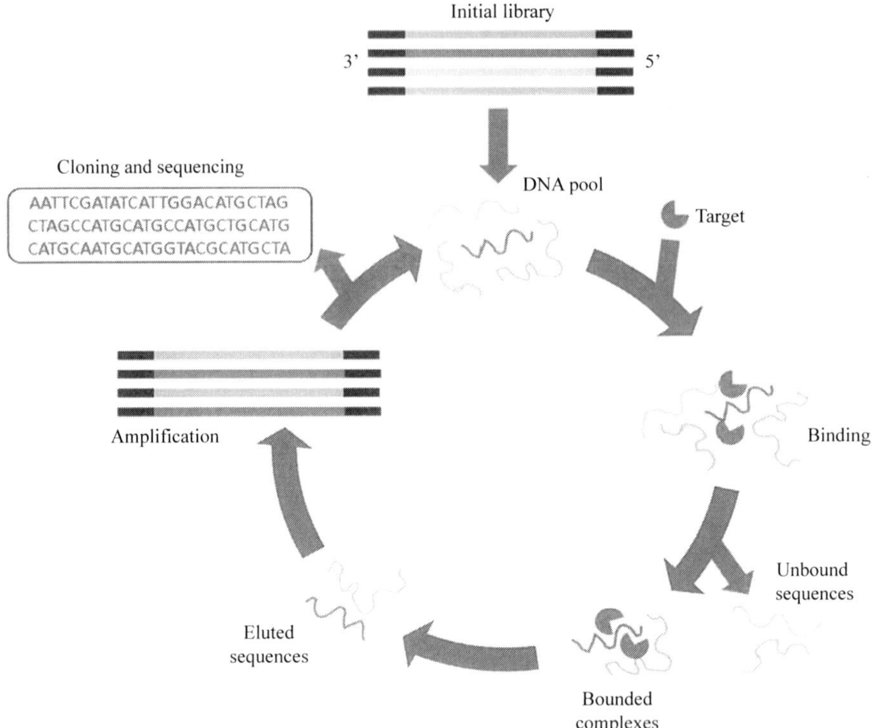

Fig. 5.2: Schematic representation of the SELEX process

Applications in the Dairy Industry

There has been a prevalence of harmful toxicants and contaminants in the dairy foods that are consumed. As these pose a great health risk, there is a dire need to mitigate such challenges. Aptamer based detection and analyses techniques can be employed in this aspect. This section summarizes some of the developments that have taken place in the field of aptamer applications on processing and safety of dairy products.

Detection of Pathogenic Microorganisms

The conventional methods used for the detection of microorganisms is the plate count method, which take log time to generate results. Aptamers can be used for such detection tests as they are quick and accurate. Aptamers can be screened by appropriate screening techniques whereby cell components or whole cell can be used as a target. Certain aptamer based sensor can even detect specific microorganisms or single colony forming unit (CFU) due to high specificity (Liu and Zhang, 2015). Usually, the aptamers are fixed by cross-linking to a slid-phase bed by one end (3' end) and the free 5' end has indicators, such as fluorescent elements (biotin), gold nanoparticle. A signal is generated when the target cell or its components bind the aptamer. In a study, He *et al.* (2014) developed a flow-cytometry assay based on aptamer-fluorescent silica nanoparticles bioconjugates for detection of *Staphylococcus aureus* in milk. The *S. aureus* cells were incubated with the aptamer nanoparticles conjugates and stained with SYBR green I dye and determined using two-color flow cytometry assay. The assay enabled the detection of cells of S. aureus as low as 7.6×10^2 cells per mL sample. In a research by Yuan *et al.* (2014) developed an aptamer based sensor for detection of *S. aureus* cells in milk. The specific aptamer was immobilized on microtiter plates using biotin, whereby the inoculated milk sample was added along with streptavidin--horseradish peroxidase conjugates. Then gold nanoparticles were added to the plates whose absorbances correlated with the concentration of *S. aureus*. The detection range was up to 10^6 CFU/mL with a detection limit of 9 CFU/mL. The results could be obtained within 4 hours. Duan *et al.* (2014), in another study, developed a method for fluorometric determination of Salmonella typhimurium cells in pasteurized milk based on graphene oxide platform. The aptamer-cell complexes release of fluorophore (5-Carboxyfluorescein) from graphene oxide whose fluorescence intensity was a function of bacterial concentration. The detection range was 1×10^3 to 1×10^8 CFU/mL sample, with a detection limit of 100 CFU/mL. In another study, Jin *et al.* (2017) developed an aptamer based detection system for *E. coli* cells. The system consisted of aptamer-gold nanoparticles conjugates. When the target cells attached to the aptamers, the fluorescence intensity is measured which gave the cell concentration. The tests were conducted for food samples like milk and showed a detection range of 5-10^6 CFU/mL with a detection limit of 3 CFU/mL. The aptasensor was able to show results in 20 minutes. Recently, Song *et al.* (2019) developed an aptamer assisted by polyethylene glycol and chitosan modified graphene oxide. The aptamers were used for quantitative analysis of *Lactobacillus casei* in fermented milk beverages giving results in the range of 10^5 to 10^9 CFU/mL. Additionally, the aptamer was able to discriminate between viable and non-viable cells using fluorescence intensity differences. Thus, the aptamers have a huge potential in the food safety analysis in dairy and food industries.

Detection of Toxins

The toxins derived from plants and microorganisms metabolic processes are considered to inflict carcinogenic and mutagenic effects on humans (Liu and Zhang, 2015). The introduction of toxin is a potential health hazard. Detection of ricin, a plant toxin obtained from castor bean plants was studied by many researchers. In a study by He *et al.* (2011), ricin detection assay based on aptamer-silver dendrite conjugates with surface-enhanced Raman scattering was used on milk and other liquid foods. The detection limit for ricin B was 100 ng/mL in milk, with analysis time <40 min. The risk of toxin can be successfully mitigated by introduction of aptamers based detection and quantification systems. The toxins from the microorganisms can be broadly grouped into two types—toxins from molds (mycotoxins), and bacterial toxins. In another research, Zengin *et al.* (2015) developed an aptamer with silver nanoparticles with 4, 4'-bipyridyl with a limit of detection of 0.32 fM for ricin B in milk and other liquid foods.

Bacterial toxins such as toxins from *Staphylococcal* endotoxins account for a large cases of food poisoning. Among the toxin, the serological type A (SEA) is most prevalent (Huang *et al.,* 2014). In a study by Huang *et al.* (2014), a magnetic bead based aptamer was fabricated with K_d of 48.57 ± 6.52 nM to detect SEA in milk samples with a detection limit of 8.7×10^{-3} µg/mL sample. Botulinum toxin, a potent neurotoxin from *Clostridium botulinum* was studied and a detection kit based on RNA aptasensor was developed (Janardhanan *et al.,* 2013). The sensor had a detection limit for 23.4 ng/mL for skimmed milk.

Mycotoxins, especially alfatoxins (AF), produced by Aspergillus genera (mainly *Aspergillus flavus* and *Aspergillus parasiticus*) of molds have been well studied and detection strategies developed which has been nicely summarized by Guo *et al.* (2020). They have listed some of the works done for detection of AF M1 in milk and milk products. Aptasensor based on carbon electrode and ferri/ferrocyanide probe was used to detect F M1 in milk (detection range 2-150 ng/L). Few fluorescent based aptasensors have been developed by the same research group to detect AF M1 in milk powders having detection range of 0.2-10 µg/kg.

Detection of Antibiotics

The presence of antibiotics has been strictly controlled and regulated by several regulated agencies like the United States Food and Drug Administration (USFDA), Codex Alimentarius Commission (CAC), European Union (EU), Food Safety and Standard Authority of India (FSSAI). Currently, the antibiotics are detected and quantified by chromatographic or immunoassay techniques. Some of the common antibiotics include streptomycin, neomycin, chloramphenicol, tetracycline etc. In a study, Jeong *et al.* (2012) developed a competitive enzyme line RNA based aptamer assay for detection of tetracycline in bovine milk. The detection range of tetracycline was reported to be 3.16×10^{-8} to 3.16×10^{-4} M. In another research, Emrani *et al.* (2016) developed a streptomycin detection kit based on DNA-gold nanoparticles conjugates. The binding of streptomycin generated fluorescence which could be measured. The observed detection limit was 47.6 nM in milk. Javidi *et al.* (2018) fabricated an aptamer-gold nanoparticles for detection of chloramphenicol in milk samples. The observed limit of detection was 0.03 nM with high specificity. Some other works on the detection of antibiotics have been discussed in detail by Liu and Zhang (2015). Thus, the antibiotic detection and quantification is a booming application of aptamer technology in dairy industries.

Detection of Allergens

Allergy due to consumption of bovine milk and dairy products is seen in infants and even some adults. The milk allergy is attributed to the protein β-lactoglobulin (β-lg), which is absent in human milk (Eissa and Zourab, 2017). Other milk proteins, like casein is also associated with milk protein allergy to little extent. In a research, Eissa and Zourab (2017) developed an aptamer based on DNA (BLG14) which had high affinity with variants of β-lg (A and B). The detection limit was 20 pg/mL with analysis time of 20 minutes. Recently, an electrochemical biosensor based on DNA/gold/$BiVO_4$ aptamer was developed by Xu *et al.* (2020) for detection of β-lg with a detection range of 0.01-1000 ng/mL.

Another novel application of aptamer technology for characterization of milk proteins and associated diseases using aptamer is the detection of β-casomorphin 7 (a peptide obtained after hydrolysis of β-casein A1). The peptide is specific to the A1 genetic variant of β-casein and leads to autism, type I diabetes, as well as heart diseases. Thus, aptamers can be used to label A1 and A2 milk (Agyei *et al.,* 2018).

Detection of Adulterants and Other Miscellaneous Compounds

Milk and dairy are prone to adulteration every now and then. Some of the common compounds that the milk is adulterated with are melamine, urea, etc. In a study, Kumar *et al.* (2015) developed an aptasensor with DNA-gold nanoparticles conjugates for detection of urea in milk samples. The DNA aptamer had K_d value of 232 nM and detection range of 20 mM to 150 mM in milk. Dong *et al.* (2016) developed a nanosensor based on thymine aptamer-modified surface-enhanced Raman scattering to detect melamine in milk.

The detection limit observed for the sensor was 1 pg/mL (1 parts per trillion) which is less than the allowed safety limit by regulatory agencies. In another study, Qiu *et al.* (2018) developed an aptasensor with evanescent wave fiber to quantitatively determine melamine in milk and infant formula. They obtained a limit of detection of 3 μM, with recovery rates of melamine from 92 to 108%.

Potential endocrine disrupting agents like like bisphenol-A have also found their way in dairy products as these are used in the packaging materials of the dairy products. Long term exposure of such compounds is detrimental to human health. Zhou *et al.* (2014) developed a label-free electrochemical aptamer based sensor for determination of bisphenol-A. The aptasensor consisted of gold nanoparticles with graphene nano composite film carbon electrode. The detection limit of bisphenol-A in milk was 0.01 μM to 10 μM with limit of detection of 5 nM.

Conclusions

Novel analytical techniques are emerging as a result of continuous research and development in science domains. Aptamer is a novel technology for food analysis and safety, whereby short single stranded DNA or RNA sequences which after suitable modification can be used for detection and quantification of several molecules. The technology has shown to have higher sensitivity and specificity than conventional antibody assays. Also, they have lower costs and quicker in nature. There has been tremendous research on use of aptamer and aptamer based sensors for the qualification and quantification of pathogenic microorganisms, toxins for bacteria, or molds, antibiotics, pesticides, adulterants etc. However, the field is still in its infancy and requires future research to broaden the scope of detection of plethora of drugs, antibiotics, emerging pathogens, adulterants and toxins. This will help in their commercialization and adoption by the food and dairy industries.

References

Agyei, D., Acquah, C., Tan, K. X., Hii, H. K., Rajendran, S. R., Udenigwe, C. C. & Danquah, M. K. (2018). Prospects in the use of aptamers for characterizing the structure and stability of bioactive proteins and peptides in food. *Analytical and Bioanalytical Chemistry*, 410(2): 297-306.

Darmostuk, M., Rimpelova, S., Gbelcova, H. & Ruml, T. (2015). Current approaches in SELEX: An update to aptamer selection technology. *Biotechnology Advances*, 33(6): 1141-1161.

Dong, N., Hu, Y., Yang, K. & Liu, J. (2016). Development of aptamer-modified SERS nanosensor and oligonucleotide chip to quantitatively detect melamine in milk with high sensitivity. *Sensors and Actuators B: Chemical*, 228: 85-93.

Dong, Y., Xu, Y., Yong, W., Chu, X. & Wang, D. (2014). Aptamer and its potential applications for food safety. *Critical Reviews in Food Science and Nutrition*, 54(12): 1548-1561.

Duan, Y. F., Ning, Y., Song, Y. & Deng, L. (2014). Fluorescent aptasensor for the determination of Salmonella typhimurium based on a graphene oxide platform. *Microchimica Acta*, 181(5-6): 647-653.

Eissa, S. & Zourob, M. (2017). In vitro selection of DNA aptamers targeting β-lactoglobulin and their integration in graphene-based biosensor for the detection of milk allergen. *Biosensors and Bioelectronics*, 91: 169-174.

Emrani, A. S., Danesh, N. M., Lavaee, P., Ramezani, M., Abnous, K. & Taghdisi, S. M. (2016). Colorimetric and fluorescence quenching aptasensors for detection of streptomycin in blood serum and milk based on double-stranded DNA and gold nanoparticles. *Food Chemistry*, 190: 115-121.

He, L., Lamont, E., Veeregowda, B., Sreevatsan, S., Haynes, C. L., Diez-Gonzalez, F. & Labuza, T. P. (2011). Aptamer-based surface-enhanced Raman scattering detection of ricin in liquid foods. *Chemical Science*, 2(8): 1579-1582.

He, X., Li, Y., He, D., Wang, K., Shangguan, J. & Shi, H. (2014). Aptamer-fluorescent silica nanoparticles bioconjugates based dual-color flow cytometry for specific detection of Staphylococcus aureus. *Journal of Biomedical Nanotechnology*, 10(7): 1359-1368.

Huang, Y., Chen, X., Xia, Y., Wu, S., Duan, N., Ma, X. & Wang, Z. (2014). Selection, identification and application of a DNA aptamer against Staphylococcus aureus enterotoxin A. *Analytical Methods*, 6(3): 690-697.

Janardhanan, P., Mello, C. M., Singh, B. R., Lou, J., Marks, J. D. & Cai, S. (2013). RNA aptasensor for rapid detection of natively folded type A botulinum neurotoxin. *Talanta*, 117: 273-280.

Javidi, M., Housaindokht, M. R., Verdian, A. & Razavizadeh, B. M. (2018). Detection of chloramphenicol using a novel apta-sensing platform based on aptamer terminal-lock in milk samples. *Analytica Chimica Acta*, 1039: 116-123.

Jeong, S. & Rhee Paeng, I. (2012). Sensitivity and selectivity on aptamer-based assay: the determination of tetracycline residue in bovine milk. *The Scientific World Journal*, 2012: 15946.

Jin, B., Wang, S., Lin, M., Jin, Y., Zhang, S., Cui, X., Gong, Y., Li, A., Xu, F. & Lu, T. J. (2017). Upconversion nanoparticles based FRET aptasensor for rapid and ultrasenstive bacteria detection. *Biosensors and Bioelectronics,* 90: 525-533.

Kumar, P., Lambadi, P. R. & Navani, N. K. (2015). Non-enzymatic detection of urea using unmodified gold nanoparticles based aptasensor. *Biosensors and Bioelectronics*, 72: 340-347.

Liu, X. & Zhang, X. (2015). Aptamer-based technology for food analysis. *Applied Biochemistry and Biotechnology*, 175(1): 603-624.

Mandal, R., Shi, Y., Singh, A., Yada, R. Y. & Singh, A. P. (2020). Food Safety and Preservation. In *Encyclopedia of Gastroenterology* (2nd ed.), E. J. Kuipers (Ed.). Academic Press, London. pp. 467-479.

Paniel, N. & Noguer, T. (2019). Detection of Salmonella in Food Matrices, from Conventional Methods to Recent Aptamer-Sensing Technologies. *Foods*, 8(9): 371.

Qiu, Y., Tang, Y., Li, B., Gu, C. & He, M. (2018). Aptamer-based detection of melamine in milk using an evanescent wave fiber sensor. *Analytical Methods*, 10(40): 4871-4878.

Rothlisberger, P., & Hollenstein, M. (2018). Aptamer chemistry. *Advanced Drug Delivery Reviews*, 134: 3-21.

Schmitz, F. R. W., Valério, A., de Oliveira, D. & Hotza, D. (2020). An overview and future prospects on aptamers for food safety. *Applied Microbiology and Biotechnology*, 104: 6929-6939.

Song, S., Wang, X., Xu, K., Ning, L. & Yang, X. (2019). Rapid identification and quantitation of the viable cells of Lactobacillus casei in fermented dairy products using an aptamer-based strategy powered by a novel cell-SELEX protocol. *Journal of Dairy Science*, 102(12): 10814-10824.

Xu, S., Dai, B., Zhao, W., Jiang, L. & Huang, H. (2020). Electrochemical detection of β-lactoglobulin based on a highly selective DNA aptamer and flower-like Au@ BiVO4 microspheres. *Analytica Chimica Acta*, 1120: 1-10.

Zengin, A., Tamer, U. & Caykara, T. (2015). Fabrication of a SERS based aptasensor for detection of ricin B toxin. *Journal of Materials Chemistry B*, 3(2): 306-315.

Zhou, L., Wang, J., Li, D. & Li, Y. (2014). An electrochemical aptasensor based on gold nanoparticles dotted graphene modified glassy carbon electrode for label-free detection of bisphenol A in milk samples. *Food Chemistry*, 162: 34-40.

6

Application and Advancement of Microbial Bio-Sensor in Food and Dairy Industry

Falguni Patra[a] and Raj Kumar Duary[b]

[a]Mansinhbhai Institute of Dairy & Food Technology, Dudhsagar Dairy Campus, Mehsana, Gujarat, India
[b]Department of Food Engineering and Technology, Tezpur University Napaam, Sonitpur, Assam, India

Abstract

Biosensors are analytical devices that use biological sensing element like enzymes, aptamer, peptides, antibody, whole cells, receptor etc. with appropriate transducer; have wide application in various fields like food pharmaceutical, medicine and other industries. Advantages of using microbial cells as biological sensing element include their low cost, easy reproduction, more resistance to change in pH and temperature and less sensitive to inhibitory substances as compared to enzymes and are suitable for genetic manipulation. Microbial sensors have been primarily developed for environmental monitoring, however for application in food and dairy industry, microbial sensors have been proposed to determine specific component of food, to detect safety parameters like antibiotics, mycotoxins, pesticides, heavy metals, to monitor fermentation processes. The chapter will focus on current knowledge on microbial biosensors, fabrication of these microbial sensors including working principle and application in food and dairy industry.

Introduction

Biosensors are the next generation detection devices, use biological sensing elements like enzymes, nucleic acids, antibody, cells, organelles, tissues, receptors; have got varied applications in the field of drug discovery, diagnosis, biomedicine, food safety and processing, environmental monitoring, defense and security etc. Microbial biosensors are analytical device that uses naturally occurring or engineered microbial cells as the recognition elements to detect physiological changes in cells with the help of suitable physicochemical transducer. Advantages of using microorganisms as biosensing element is their rapid growth, easy to culture, comparatively easy for genetic manipulation, low cost and microorganisms metabolize range of chemicals. In addition to this, microbes are more tolerant of pH and temperature and less sensitive to inhibitory substances when compared to enzymes (Nakamura, 2018). Mainly bacteria like *Escherichia coli, Gluconobacter oxydans, Pseudomonas alcaligenes, Ps. Fluorescens, Shewanella oneidensis, Methylobacterium organophilium, Acaligense* spp., *Streptococcus thermophillus, Lactobacillus* spp., *Bacillus sphaericus, B. badius, Raoultella terrigena, Microbacterium phyllosphaerae* etc. and yeasts like *Saccharomyces cerevisiae, Arxula adeninivorans, Kluyveromyces fragilis, Kluyveromyces marxianus, Hansenula polymorpha, Trichosporon cutaneum, Pichia pastoris, Candida tropicalis* have used for development of microbial biosensors. Bacteriophages also have been used as biosensing element to develop biosensor mainly to detect pathogens.

Living microorganism when used as biosensing element in microbial biosensors, are based on either inhibition of microbial respiration by the components of interest like heavy metals, toxins etc. or based on metabolism of cells i.e., substrate assimilation of microorganism is used as index of metabolic activity (Xu and Ying, 2011). However, when dead microbial cells are used, the analysis is based on extracellular or intracellular enzymes which the microorganism contains and the reactions catalyzed by them. Microorganisms also have been genetically modified mainly for better sensitivity and selectivity. Bacteria have been genetically engineered to respond against stresses (physiological or chemical) through the synthesis of a reporter protein e.g., luciferase, green fluorescent protein (GFP), or β-galactosidase. However, luminescent bacteria naturally present have also been used for development of microbial biosensors.

Microbial biosensors can be classified based on the sensor system i.e., flow or batch, can be either electrochemical or bioluminescence based on signal type and either analyte specific or non-specific.

Till now, microbial biosensors have been developed for analytes like heavy metals and metalloids (As, Cd, Zn, Ni, Cu, Cr, Cu), organic xenobiotics such as naphthalene, benzene, toluene, ethylbenzene, xylene, alkylsulphonates, polychlorinated biphenyls, various nutrients and physiologically active molecules. In the dairy and food industry, microbial biosensors have been applied for determination of various components of foods like sugars, short-chain fatty acids, amino acids, or vitamins, metabolizable products like e.g. ethanol, urea etc., to detect pathogens and their toxins and to monitor antibiotics, pesticides and heavy metals etc. (Table 6.1). In the fermented food category, microbial biosensors also have been applied for monitoring fermentation process. Application of Microbial Biosensors in Food and Dairy Industry.

Food quality and safety is major concern worldwide and analysis of food products held great importance to ensure that. Biosensors being the next generation analytical device are promising option for food and dairy industry. Microbial biosensors have been applied to determine specific nutritional components in food, for bioprocess monitoring in food fermentation, to detect component which affect safety of the food products and to measure and monitor BOD of food and dairy industry waste water.

Analysis of Carbohydrate

L-rhamnose-inducible microbial biosensor was developed by Lukasiak *et al.* (2012) for analysis of pectin using engineered *E. coli* in which P_{rhaB} promoter was fused with promoter less *luxCDABE* genes of *Vibrio fischeri* within plasmid pUCD615. The microbial sensor determined L-rhamnose in the pectin samples of citrus peel, orange peel, apple and sugar beet pulp in the range 15 and 10 mmol/L with a response time of 60 min. Previously a hybrid biosensor with *Saccharomyces cerevisiae,* glucose oxidase and catalase and potentiometric oxygen electrode was reported for analysis of sucrose in presence of glucose. The developed sensor determined sucrose linearly in the range 1×10^{-5} to 3×10^{-2} M and was used for sucrose estimation in soft drinks (Rotariu *et al.,* 2002). For monitoring glucose and maltose in food manufacturing and fermentation process, Liu *et al.* (2017) constructed biosensor by immobilizing glucoamylase-displayed bacteria and glucose dehydrogenase-displayed bacteria on multi-walled carbon nanotubes (MWNTs) modified glassy carbon electrode (GCE). The developed sensor determined glucose and maltose in the range 0.1-2.0 mM and 0.2-10 mM, with limit of detection (LOD) of 0.04 mM and 0.1 mM, respectively.

Table 6.1: Application of microbial biosensors in dairy and food industries

Analyte	Microorganism used	LOD	Linear detection range	Application in foods	Reference
L-rhamnose	Engineered *E. coli*		15 and 10 mmol /L	Citrus peel, orange peel, apple and sugar beet pulp	Lukasiak et al (2012)
Sucrose	*Saccharomyces cerevisiae*		1×10^{-5} to 3×10^{-2} M	Soft drinks	Rotariu et al (2002)
Glucose and maltose	Glucoamylase-displayed bacteria and glucose dehydrogenase-displayed bacteria	0.04mM and 0.1mM respectively	0.1-2.0mM and 0.2-10mM respectively		Liu et al (2017)
L-ascorbic acid	*Candida tropicalis*	62 μM (amperometric) and 59 μM (DPV)	100 and 1500 μM	Orange, lemon, grape fruit and in two types of Vit C tablet	Akyilmaz et al(2020)
Ethanol	*Methylobacterium organophilium*	0.025 mM	0.050–7.5 mM	Wine samples	Wen et al (2013)
Lactic acid and pyruvic acid	lyophilised cells of *Lactobacillus delbruecki*	0.012 mM for lactate , 0.018 mM for pyruvate	0.1 and 1.0 mM	Milk, butter milk, kefir	Canbay et al (2015)
Caffeine	*Pseudomonas alcaligenes*		0.1 to 1 mg /mL	Instant tea , coffee	Babu et al (2007)
Phenol	*Acaligense sp.*		0.5–5.0 mM and 0.7–10 mM	Red wine	Kim et al (2011)
Catechol	*Lactobacillus spp., Streptococcus thermophilus*		0.5 and 5.0 m*M*	Milk products	Sagiroglu et al (2011)
Riboflavin	*Shewanella oneidensis*	2.2 nM	5 nM - 10 μM		Si et al 2016)

Analyte	Microorganism used	LOD	Linear detection range	Application in foods	Reference
Arginine	*Hansenula polymorpha*	0.085 mM	Till 0.6 mM	Wine, juice samples	Stasyuk et al (2014)
L-lysine	*S. cerevisiae*		1.0 and 10.0 µM		Akyilmaz et al (2007)
Estrogenic mycotoxin	Engineered *S. cerevisiae*			Spiked milk samples	Valimaa et al (2010)
Nisin	Genetically engineered *Lactococcus lactis*	1 ng/mL		Milk	Landete et al (2020)
Tetracycline , oxytetracycline	Engineered *E. coli*		10-60 ng /mL and 25-125 ng/ mL respectively	Goat milk	Scaria et al (2009)
Ciprofloxacin	Engineered *E. coli*	8 ng/mL in milk, egg white, chicken essence, and 64 ng/ mL for egg yolk		Milk , egg white, and chicken essence	Kao et al (2018)
Ciprofloxacin	Engineered *E. coli*	7.2 ng/mL		Whole milk	Lu et al (2019)
Methanol	*Methylobacterium organophilium*	0.047 mM	0.050–2.5 mM	Apple juice	Wen et al (2014)
Ni(II)	*Bacillus sphaericus*		0.002–0.04 ppb	Wheat flour	Verma and Singh (2006)
Cadmium	Engineered *E. coli*	5 µg/L	10–50 µg/L	Milk	Kumar et al (2017)
Lead	*B. sphaericus*	$2.4*10^{-3}$ nM		Milk	Verma et al (2011)
Lead	*B. sphaericus*		10-1000 µg/L	Milk	Verma et al (2016)
Organophosphorus pesticides	Engineered *E. coli*	1×10^{-9} M		Apple	Khatun et al (2018)
ethanol for fermentation monitoring	*Gluconobacter oxydans*	5 µM	10 µM - 1 mM		Šefčovičová et al (2012)

Analyte	Microorganism used	LOD	Linear detection range	Application in foods	Reference
2-phenylethanol	*G. oxydans*	1mM	0.02–0.70 mM	Phenylacetic acid bioproduction	Schenkmayerová et al (2015)
Salmonella typhimurium	*Bacteriophage*	5×10^3 CFU/mL		Fat free milk	Lakshmanan et al (2007)
Escherichia coli O157:H7, *E. coli* O45:H2	*Bacteriophage*	10–50 CFU/mL		Spinach, ground beef and chicken homogenates	Anany et al. (2018)
BOD7	*E. coli* R17.1.3 and *Raoultella terrigena*		5–200 mg/ L and 50 mg /L	Dairy waste water	Raud et al (2010)
BOD	*Microbacterium phyllosphaerae*			Dairy waste water	Kibena et al (2013)

Analysis of L-Ascorbic acid

L-Ascorbic acid (L-AA) i.e., vitamin C have important biological role such as enhancing immunity, prevention of cancer, free radical metabolism etc. As a result vitamin C is used as antioxidant in variety of foods, pharmaceutical preparation and in cosmetics. Thus, there is a need of appropriate analytical methods for determination of L-Ascorbic acid. First Vit C microbial sensor was designed by Akyilmaz et al. (2020) with *Candida tropicalis* based on conversion of L-Ascorbic acid to dehydro-L-Ascorbic acid (by ascorbate oxidase) by *C. tropicalis* yeast cells. The biosensor was fabricated by immobilizing lyophilized *C. tropicalis* yeast cells with o-aminophenol on a platinum electrode surface by electropolymerization and amperometry and differential pulse voltammetry (DPV) was used for quantification of Vit C. L - Ascorbic acid was determined in the range 100 and 1500 µM, with detection limit (LOD) of 62 µM (amperometric) and 59 µM (DPV) and response time was 14 s (DPV) and 5 s (amperometric). The developed biosensor was applied for L - Ascorbic acid determination in orange, lemon, grape fruit and in two types of Vit C tablet and author concluded that microbial biosensor determined L - Ascorbic acid quantitatively and more accurately as compared to DCIP reference method (Akyilmaz *et al.*, 2020).

Analysis of Ethanol

Rotariu *et al.* (2004) proposed a potentiometric oxygen electrode based biosensor using *Saccharomyces ellipsoideus,* the sensor measured ethanol in 7 min for the steady-state method and 2 min for kinetic measurements. *C. tropicalis* cells based amperometric ethanol biosensor was reported by Akyilmaz and Dinçkaya, (2005) which detected ethanol in the range 0.5 and 7.5 mM within response time of 2 min. *M. organophilium* based microbial sensor for detection of ethanol in wine samples was reported by Wen *et al.* (2013). The developed sensor detected ethanol linearly in the range 0.050–7.5 mM with LOD of 0.025 mM and response time 100 sec. The microbial sensor was applied for ethanol determination in various alcohol samples and results were comparable to the gas chromatographic method.

Analysis of Lactic Acid

Concentration of lactic acid is important parameter in determining quality of various foods and beverages and appropriate analytical methods are thus necessary. Chen and Jin, (2011) reported about an amperometric microbial biosensor for sensitive determination of lactic acid. The sensor was developed by co-immobilizing *Lb. bulgaricus* and *S. thermophilus* on the surface of oxygen electrode. The resultant sensor determined lactate in the range 0 to 300 μmol/ L with a sensitivity of 1.87 mA mol/ L and response time of 240 s. Canbay *et al.* (2015) proposed an amperometric microbial biosensor for simultaneous determination of lactic acid and pyruvic acid based on lyophilized cells of *Lb. delbruecki* and used the biosensor for lactic acid determination in samples of milk, kefir and buttermilks. The sensor was fabricated by immobilizing *Lb. delbruecki* cells with polypyrrole on a platin electrode surface using electropolymerization. The developed sensor determined lactic acid and pyruvic acid linearly in the range 0.1 and 1.0 mM with LOD 0.012 mM for lactate and 0.018 mM for pyruvate within response time of 3 sec.

Analysis of Caffeine

Caffeine is naturally present in coffee, cocoa beans, cola nuts and tea leaves and is a mild stimulant and has therapeutic values. However, as it is stimulant, its excess consumption has adverse effects on human health particularly pregnant women and elderly people. Coffee being one of the popular beverages worldwide, its caffeine content is a measure of quality for different types of coffee beverages. Babu *et al.* (2007) used caffeine degrading *Pseudomonas alcaligenes* MTCC 5264 to construct an amperometric biosensor for detection of caffeine in solutions. The biosensor was fabricated by immobilizing whole cells of *Ps. Alcaligenes* MTCC 5264 onto cellophane membrane; as crosslinking agent and protein based stabilizing agent glutaraledhyde and gelatin was used respectively. The developed sensor identified caffeine in the range 0.1 to 1 mg/ mL within response time of 3 min and was applied for caffeine determination in instant tea and coffee samples; the results were in good correlation with HPLC. The author also stated that the developed microbial sensor was specific for caffeine and there was negligible response for interfering compounds like theophylline, theobromine, paraxanthine, other methyl xanthines and sugars.

Analysis of Phenol

Phenolic compounds are regarded as good antioxidants, are naturally present in various foods like fruits, vegetables, nuts, seeds etc. A microbial sensor was proposed by Kim *et al.* (2011) by immobilizing *Acaligense spp.* on the surface of glassy carbon electrode coupled with CdS-MWNT and Cu2S-MWNT (quantum dot-modified multi-wall carbon nanotube QD-MWNT) composites. The detection range for CdS-MWNT and Cu2S-MWNT based biosensor were 0.5–5.0 mM and 0.7–10 mM for phenol respectively. The developed senor was used for phenol estimation in commercial red wine samples. Different forms of *Lactobacillus spp* was used for development of microbial biosensor for determination of phenolic compounds in milk and milk products. Freeze died cells of *Lactobacilli* (containing *Lb. bulgaricus, Lb. acidophilus,*

Streptococcus thermophilus), pure *Lb. acidophilus*, pure *Lb. bulgaricus*, and *Lb. acidophilus*- and *Lb. bulgaricus* adapted to catechol in MRS broth was immobilized in gelatin by using glutaraldehyde. The developed biosensor determined catechol within response time of 18 min in the range 0.5 and 5.0 m*M* and was applied for determination of phenolic compounds in milk products (Sagiroglu *et al.,* 2011). A genetically engineered *E. coli* displaying laccase on the cell surface was immobilized onto a glassy-carbon electrode for biosensing catechol. The developed electrochemical sensor responded linearly to catechol in the range 0.5 μM–300.0 μM with LOD 0.1 μM. Red wine and tea samples were analyzed in the biosensor and a recovery rate of 98.2%–103.8% was determined. The researchers also reported that the biosensor showed good stability, reproducibility and its performance was comparable with HPLC (Zhang *et al.,* 2018).

Analysis of Riboflavin

An amperometric microbial biosensor based on *Shewanella oneidensis* MR-1 was proposed for riboflavin determination in food, pharmaceutical, and clinical samples employing "bioelectrochemical wire" (BW) composed of riboflavin and cytochrome C between *S. oneidensis* MR-1 and electrode. The developed microbial senor determined riboflavin linearly in the range 5 nM - 10 μM with a LOD 2.2 nM (Si *et al.,* 2016). Another whole-cell electrochemical sensor was developed by Yu *et al.* (2017) for determination of riboflavin content in food and pharmaceutical samples employing whole-cell based riboflavin redox cycling system. The researchers have used electroactive bacteria *S. oneidensis* MR-1 as a biocatalyst for regeneration of the reduced riboflavin after the electrode oxidation. The developed amperometric sensor showed LOD 0.85 ± 0.09 nM with great selectivity and stability.

Analysis of Amino Acid

Arginine

Analysis of arginine concentration is used as a quality control parameter for fermented foods, beverages, wine and other food supplements as at high concentration, arginine is converted into ethyl carbamate during fermentation (Verma *et al.,* 2017). An amperometric biosensor for analysis of L-arginine was reported based of recombinant methylotrophic yeast *Hansenula polymorpha* (Stasyuk *et al.,* 2014). The sensor was fabricated by co-immobilization of *H. polymorpha* cells and commercial urease onto the surface of electrode. The resultant microbial biosensor detected L-arginine linearly till 0.6 mM Arg with LOD 0.085 mM, sensitivity 14±1.2 A (M/m^2) in the response time 60 sec and was applied for L-arginine analysis in wine and juice samples.

L-lysine

L-lysine is an essential amino acid, present in mostly animal foods sources, lysine content is related to protein quality of foods and used as an indicator for effects of industrial processes or during cooking treatment. *S. cerevisiae* NRRL-12632 was used for development of amperometric microbial biosensor for determination of L-lysine amino acid (based on lysine oxidase). L-lysine was determined based on the differences of the respiration *S. cerevisiae* NRRL-12632 cells on the oxygen meter in the absence and the presence of L-lysine. The developed biosensor determined L-lysine linearly in the range 1.0 and 10.0 μM with 1 min response time (Akyilmaz *et al.,* 2007).

Determination of Mycotoxin

Mycotoxins produced by various fungi like the *Aspergillus, Penicillium*, and *Fusarium* enter food chain through mainly contaminated food and feed. Fungal toxin like aflatoxin, ochratoxins, zearalanone etc. are known to cause estrogenic, gastrointestinal, and kidney disorders, mutations and cancers. A bioluminescent microbial biosensor with genetically engineered *S. cerevisiae* to produce firefly luciferase-enzyme was developed for determination estrogenic mycotoxin residues in milk. The sensor detected mycotoxins in nanomolar concentration in less than 3 hrs assay time in the milk samples spiked with zearalanone, α-zearalanol, β-zearalanol, α-zearalenol and β-zearalenol (Valimaa *et al.,* 2010).

Determination of Nisin

Nisin is an bacteriocin, currently approved by EU for application as an additive (biopreservative) in ripened and processed cheese, clotted cream, puddings such as semolina or tapioca, mascarpone, and pasteurized liquid egg and in US, Australia, New Zealand and other countries nisin is approved for use in various foods like sauces, soups, salads, dressings, and ready-to-eat and processed meat products etc. Recently a whole cell nisin biosensor was reported by Landete *et al.* (2020) for determining nisin in milk and colonic model using genetically engineered *Lactococcus lactis* strain. The strain was transformed with the vector with two bioreporters pNZ:Nis-aFP or pNZ:Nis-mCherry, that encoded for the anaerobic fluorescent protein evoglow-Pp1 (aFP) or the fluorescent protein mCherry. The biosensor detected nisin produced by *L. lactis* INIA 650 in milk. The researcher found that reporter system pNZ:Nis-mCherry had higher sensibility, detected nisin concentrations of 1 ng/mL produced by *L.lactis* INIA 650 in colonic media as determined by agar diffusion or cross streak bioassays.

Detection of Antibiotics

Veterinary drugs such as β -lactam, tetracycline, amino glycoside, sulfonamide and macrolides are commonly used for the treatment of various diseases like mastitis, brucellosis etc. Presence of these antibiotics in milk and other animal foods has adverse effect including allergic reaction in susceptible consumer and development of multi drug resistance pathogens. EU has set maximum residue limits (MRLs) for antibiotics in food products of animal origin to protect consumer health. Virolainen *et al.* (2008) developed a microbial biosensor with *E. coli* strain harbouring a plasmid containing a bacterial luciferase operon under the control of a tetracycline sensitive repressor (lux operon was induced and bioluminescent signal was produced only in presence of tetracycline) for determination of tetracyclines and their 4-epimer derivatives in poultry meat. The same biosensor was later used for screening more than 300 routine poultry samples and the results were compared with a microbial inhibition test. The researchers reported that microbial biosensor assay was more accurate than inhibition test which exhibited 10.2% suspected samples compared to 2% by inhibition test which was confirmed by liquid chromatography-tandem mass spectrometry (LC-MS/MS) (Pikkemaat *et al.,* 2010). A genetically modified *E. coli* JM109 (pJSKV41) was used for development of whole cell based biosensor for detection of tetracyclines in milk and water samples (Scaria *et al.,* 2009). The strain was modified with a plasmid containing a transcriptional fusion between tetR regulated tet promoter and Enhanced Green Fluorescent Protein (EGFP) gene. The developed biosensor detected tetracycline in the range of 10-60 ng /mL and oxytetracycline in the range of 25-125 ng/ mL; the author also reported that residual tetracycline content in goat milk was determined after 4 days of tetracycline treatment. A genetically live bacteria biosensor was integrated into a CCD-based lens-free optical analyzer (LumiSense) for rapid, simple, sensitive and high through put detection of antibiotics. The microbial biosensor based on *E. coli* RFM strain which harbored a fusion of the *E.coli* recA gene promoter to the Photorhabdus luminescens luxCDABE bioluminescence gene cassette, was used for determination of ciprofloxacin in samples of milk, egg white, and chicken essence. The author demonstrated that the developed sensor could detect ciprofloxacin between 20 and 80 min with LOD 8 ng/mL in milk, egg white, and chicken essence, and 64 ng/mL for egg yolk (Kao *et al.,* 2018). Lu *et al.* (2019) reported about an integral smart phone-based whole-cell biosensor LumiCellSense (LCS) with bioluminescent *E. coli* bioreporter cells for detection of ciprofloxacin. The reporter cell emitted luminescence in presence of target chemical which was then imaged by camera, and a dedicated phone-embedded application, LCS_Logger. The developed sensing system was applied for determination of ciprofloxacin (CIP), in whole milk, and showed LOD of 7.2 ng/mL.

Analysis of Methanol

Methanol when consumed metabolize into formic acid and/ or formate salts which are poisonous for our central nervous system and may result into blindness, coma, and death. Wen *et al.* (2014) reported about a microbial biosensor composed of gold nanoparticles immobilized eggshell membrane, an oxygen sensor with *M. organophilium* for determination of methanol. The biosensor analysed methanol linearly in the range 0.050–2.5 mM with LOD of 0.047 mM and response time of less than 60 s. Methanol content of the apple juice was analyzed by the developed sensor and the results were comparable with gas chromatographic method. The working principle of biosensor was based on respiration of *M. organophilium* cells i.e. dissolved oxygen consumption in presence of methanol in the samples.

Detection of Heavy Metals

Heavy metals are abundantly present in the environment and have toxic effects on human health. Long time exposure of heavy metals even in low concentration have potential detrimental effect and are known to cause genotoxicity, carcinogenesis of intestine, lung, ovary, metabolic disorders and disruption central nervous system (Bae *et al.*, 2018). Heavy metals may leach into food products from environment and thus monitoring heavy metals is used as a quality and safety parameter for foods.

Ni (II)

Verma and Singh, (2006) reported about a microbial biosensor for measuring Ni(II) using *B. sphaericus* MTCC 5100 secreting urease enzyme and applied for analysis of Ni(II) in wheat flour. An NH^{4+} ion selective electrode along with potentiometer was used as a transducer and the resultant biosensor detected Ni(II) in the range 0.002–0.04 ppb with in response time of 1.5 minutes.

Cadmium

Cadmium is the seventh most toxic substance according to the list of toxic substances named as "Top 20 hazardous substances" released by Agency for Toxic Substances and Disease Registry. *B. badius* cells was used for development of electrochemical biosensor for detection of cadmium based on urease inhibition (Verma *et al.*, 2011). The biosensor was fabricated by immobilizing *B. badius* cells onto the nylon membranes and sol-gel method was applied with alcohol and Tetra Ethyl Ortho Silicate. The resultant microbial biosensor was used for Cd determination in raw milk and spiked milk samples. For detection of cadmium, a whole cell biosensor was developed using genetically engineered *E. coli* DH5α (pNV12) with *gfp* gene under the control of *cad* promoter and the *cadC* gene of *Staphylococcus aureus* plasmid pI258. The sensor determined cadmium in the range 10–50 μg/L with LOD of 10 μg/L within 15 min; the LOD can be reduced upto 5 μg/L with 30 min incubation. The sensor was also converted into a miniature microarray format and was successfully used for detection of cadmium in milk (Kumar *et al.,* 2017).

Lead

Elemental and inorganic lead components has been classified as portable human carcinogen by EPA. Verma *et al.* (2011) reported about a whole cell lead biosensor by immobilizing urease producing *B. sphaericus* (MTCC5100) on the surface of carbon paste electrode and unutilized NADPH oxidation was used to measure the lead concentration in the sample. Milk samples were specifically pre concentrated using lead specific column and detection limit of 2.4×10^{-3} nM was achieved which is below the permissible limit of lead in milk. A disposable optical biosensor for lead detection was developed by Verma *et al.* (2016). The sensor was fabricated immobilizing urease producing *B. sphaericus* and phenol red in the glass capillary (act as a microchannel) using sol-gel approach and calcium alginate. The assay was based on the inhibition of urease in presence of lead. The biosensor showed linearity in the range of 10-1000 μg/L, require I ml sample for analysis and can be used in milk samples with minimum modification.

Analysis of Pesticides

Pesticides like organophosphorus pesticides (OPPs), organo chlorine pesticide (OCPs), pyrethroids and carbamates may gain entry into food and animal feeds as they are very commonly used in agricultural farms to control pests. Upon consumption, pesticides may be metabolized, excreted, stored, or bioaccumulated in body fat and has adverse effect on human health including neurological, dermatological, gastrointestinal, carcinogenic, respiratory, reproductive and endocrine effects (Nicolopoulou-Stamati *et al*., 2016). Biosensors have been developed to monitor pesticide residues in food industry. For on-site monitoring of p-nitrophenyl-substituted organophosphates (OPs) compounds, a microbial biosensor was proposed utilizing genetically engineered *E. coli* displaying organophosphorus hydrolase on its surface and glass carbon electrode modified with ordered mesopore carbons. The developed biosensor exhibited linearity in the range 0.05–25 μM for paraoxon, 0.05–25 μM for parathion, and 0.08–30 μM for methyl parathion and LOD of 9.0 nM for paraoxon, 10 nM for parathion and 15 nM for methyl parathion (Tang *et al.,* 2014). Khatun *et al.* (2018) developed microbial biosensor for detection of organophosphorus pesticides using two genetically engineered *E. coli* strains; one strain hydrolyzed OPs to p-nitrophenol (PNP) and the second strain converted PNP signal into β-galactosidase production for colorimetric detection (Figure 6.1). The developed sensor could detect commonly used OPs, agriculture, detected ethyl-paraoxon @1×10^{-9} M within 3.5 h. The paper based format of the developed sensor was also applied for on-site detection of OPs in apples samples.

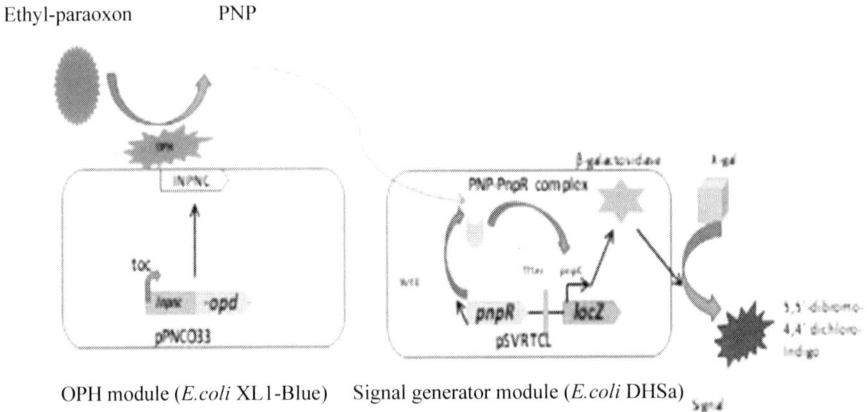

Fig. 6.1: Microbial biosensor for detection of organophosphorus pesticides

Analysis of Urea

Verma and Singh, (2003) developed a microbial biosensor using urease producing *Bacillus* spp. isolated from soil along with the ammonium ion selective electrode of a potentiometric transducer. The developed microbial sensor detected urea in milk samples within 2 min and results showed good correlation with the pure enzyme system.

Detection of Food Borne Pathogens

As bacteriophages are strain specific when infecting bacteria, this makes them ideal candidate as biocontrol agent for bacteria particularly pathogens. Lakshmanan *et al.* (2007) reported about a bacteriophage based magneto elastic sensor for the detection of *Salmonella typhimurium* in fat free milk with detection limit of 5×10^3 CFU/mL. A bacteriophage based electrochemiluminescent (ECL) biosensor was proposed for label-free detection of *Pseudomonas aeruginosa* in milk with recovery rate of 78.6% to 114.3%. The developed biosensor detected *Ps. aeruginosa* within 30 min in the range $1.4 \times 10^2 – 1.4 \times 10^6$ CFU/mL with LOD 56 CFU/mL (Yue *et al.*, 2017). Anany *et al.* (2018) reported about a paper based dipstick format with piezoelectric inkjet printing for detection of *E. coli* O157:H7, *E. coli* O45:H2, and *Salmonella newport* in spinach, ground beef and chicken homogenates along with quantitative real-time PCR to detect the progeny phages. The developed biosensor was cost effective with LOD 10–50 CFU/mL.

Application of Microbial Biosensor in Bioprocess Monitoring

Microbial biosensors have been constructed for motoring food fermentation processes like in ethanol fermentation, phenylacetic acid production etc. Valach *et al.* (2009) reported about a microbial biosensor in a flow injection analysis (FIA) system using *Gluconobacter oxydans* immobilized on the surface of combined (glassy carbon vs. Ag/AgCl) electrode. The amperometric sensor detected ethanol linearly in the range 10 μM to 1.5 mM with response time up to 3 min. The developed biosensor FIA system was applied for off-line monitoring of ethanol production during alcoholic fermentation and result showed good correlation with gas chromatography (GC) reference method. Another microbial biosensor was reported for ethanol analysis of fermentation sample was reported by Sefcovicova *et al.* (2012) based on *G. oxydans* cells. The sensor was constructed from bionanocomposite made by direct mixing of *G. oxydans* cells and carbon nanotubes and as a mediator ferricyanide was used. The developed sensor determined ethanol in the range 10 μM – 1 mM with LOD 5 μM. These authors also tested different carbon nanoparticles immobilizing same bacteria for ethanol biosensor, out of those single- or multi-walled carbon nanotubes provided the highest sensitivity of detection of 117–121 μA/ cm^2/mM. However, Ketjen black 300 and 600 provided LOD of 2–6 μM and with short response time 14–33 s and sensitivity of 84–88 μA /cm^2/mM (Sefcovicova *et al.,* 2015). Phenylacetic acid (PA) is used as a flavor (have honey like flavor at low concentration) in food industry. PA bioproduction starts with conversion of L-phenylalanine to 2-phenylethanol (2-PE) by yeast and then conversion of 2-PE to PA by acetic acid bacteria. For monitoring 2-PE for production of PA, an amperometric biosensor was developed using *G. oxydans* (immobilized within a disposable polyelectrolyte complex gel membrane composed of sodium alginate, cellulose sulphate and poly (methylene-co-guanidine) and a Clark oxygen electrode. The microbial sensor determined 2-PE (based on change in oxygen concentration) linearly in the range 0.02–0.70 mM with sensitivity of 864 nA/ mM and LOD 1mM. The biosensor had excellent storage stability and was applied for off line monitoring 2-PE biooxidation into phenylacetic acid (PA), results of which showed good correlation with gas chromatography (Schenkmayerova *et al.*, 2015).

Application of Microbial Biosensor for BOD Measurement

Live cells of *E. coli* R17.1.3 and *Raoultella terrigena* P74.3 was used for development of a semi-specific BOD biosensor by immobilizing the cells on agarose gel matrix. The sensor measured BOD7 linearly in the range 5–200 mg/ L and 50 mg /L for *R. terrigena* and *E. coli* based biosensor respectively. When evaluated for measurement of BOD7 value of dairy industry waste water, the current semi-specific biosensor overestimate the BOD7 value as compared to a reference *Ps. fluorescens* biosensor which underestimate the BOD value (Raud *et al.*, 2010). Kibena *et al.* (2013) fabricated a semi specific microbial biosensor using *Microbacterium phyllosphaerae* for monitoring BOD in dairy waste water. The developed sensor was more sensitive towards waste water containing milk solids and determined BOD of dairy waste water and butter whey by underestimating the actual BOD by 25–32%. However, when compared with a universal microbial biosensor based on *Ps. fluorescens*, the developed biosensor was better as the universal sensor based on *Ps. fluorescens* underestimate the actual BOD value by 46–61%.

Conclusions

Microbial sensors have been developed for ensuring food quality and safety by analyzing various quality and safety parameters, and for monitoring food processes. Microbial biosensors also have been miniaturized to make it portable for onsite monitoring of analytes, some were also made into dipstick version for low cost analysis and easy handling. However, their applications in food and dairy is rather limited as microbial biosensor suffers from issues like lower sensitivity, lower selectivity, lower storage life and higher response time as opposed to enzyme biosensors. Although, genetic engineering have been done to solve the problems such as poor sensitivity and selectivity, still further work is needed in the direction of developing fast, new reporter for better expression, systems for multianalyte detection, array based systems for high throughput analysis to make microbial biosensor as a commercially feasible analytical device for food and dairy industry.

References

Akyilmaz, E. & Dinçkaya, E. (2005). An amperometric microbial biosensor development based on *Candida tropicalis* yeast cells for sensitive determination of ethanol. *Biosensors and Bioelectronics*, 20(7): 1263-1269.

Akyilmaz, E., Erdogan, A., Ozturk, R. & Yasa, I. (2007). Sensitive determination of L-lysine with a new amperometric microbial biosensor based on *Saccharomyces cerevisiae* yeast cells. *Biosensors and Bioelectronics*, 22(6): 1055-1060.

Akyilmaz, E., Guvenc, C. & Koylu, H. (2020). A novel microbial biosensor system based on *C. tropicalis* yeast cells for selective determination of L-Ascorbic acid. *Bioelectrochemistry*, 132: 107420.

Anany, H., Brovko, L., El Dougdoug, N. K., Sohar, J., Fenn, H., Alasiri, N., Jabrane, T., Mangin, P., Ali, M. M., Kannan, B. & Filipe, C. D. (2018). Print to detect: a rapid and ultrasensitive phage-based dipstick assay for foodborne pathogens. *Analytical and Bioanalytical Chemistry*, *410*(4), pp.1217-1230.

Babu, V. S., Patra, S., Karanth, N. G., Kumar, M. A. & Thakur, M. S. (2007). Development of a biosensor for caffeine. *Analytica Chimica Acta*, 582(2): 329-334.

Bae, J., Lim, J. W. & Kim, T. (2018). Reusable and storable whole-cell microbial biosensors with a microchemostat platform for in situ on-demand heavy metal detection. *Sensors and Actuators B: Chemical*, 264:372-381.

Canbay, E., Habip, A., Kara, G., Eren, Z. & Akyilmaz, E. (2015). A microbial biosensor based on *Lactobacillus delbruecki* sp. bacterial cells for simultaneous determination of lactic and pyruvic acid. *Food Chemistry*, 169: 197-202.

Chen, J. & Jin, Y. (2011). Sensitive lactate determination based on acclimated mixed bacteria and palygorskite co-modified oxygen electrode. *Bioelectrochemistry*, 80(2):151-154.

Kao, W. C., Belkin, S. & Cheng, J. Y. (2018). Microbial biosensing of ciprofloxacin residues in food by a portable lens-free CCD-based analyzer. *Analytical and Bioanalytical Chemistry*, 410(4): 1257-1263.

Khatun, M. A., Hoque, M. A., Zhang, Y., Lu, T., Cui, L., Zhou, N. Y. & Feng, Y. (2018). Bacterial consortium-based sensing system for detecting organophosphorus pesticides. *Analytical Chemistry*, 90(17): 10577-10584.

Kibena, E., Raud, M., Jogi, E. & Kikas, T. (2013). Semi-specific *Microbacterium phyllosphaerae*-based microbial sensor for biochemical oxygen demand measurements in dairy wastewater. *Environmental Science and Pollution Research*, 20(4): 2492-2498.

Kim, S. K., Kwen, H. D. & Choi, S. H. (2011). Fabrication of a microbial biosensor based on QD-MWNT supports by a one-step radiation reaction and detection of phenolic compounds in red wines. *Sensors*, 11(2): 2001-2012.

Kumar, S., Verma, N. and Singh, A.K. (2017). Development of cadmium specific recombinant biosensor and its application in milk samples. *Sensors and Actuators B: Chemical*, 240: 248-254.

Lakshmanan, R. S., Guntupalli, R., Hu, J., Petrenko, V. A., Barbaree, J. M. & Chin, B. A. (2007). Detection of Salmonella typhimurium in fat free milk using a phage immobilized magnetoelastic sensor. *Sensors and Actuators B: Chemical*, *126*(2), pp.544-550.

Landete, J. M., Langa, S., Escudero, C. & Arqus, J. L. (2020). Fluorescent detection of nisin by genetically modified *Lactococcus lactis* strains in milk and a colonic model: Application of whole-cell nisin biosensors. *Journal of Bioscience and Bioengineering*, 129(4): 435-440.

Liu, A., Lang, Q., Liang, B. & Shi, J. (2017). Sensitive detection of maltose and glucose based on dual enzyme-displayed bacteria electrochemical biosensor. *Biosensors and Bioelectronics*, 87: 25-30.

Lu, M. Y., Kao, W. C., Belkin, S. & Cheng, J. Y. (2019). A Smartphone-Based Whole-Cell Array Sensor for Detection of Antibiotics in Milk. *Sensors*, 19(18): 3882.

Lukasiak, J., Georgiou, C. A., Olsen, K. & Georgakopoulos, D. G. (2012). Development of an L-rhamnose bioluminescent microbial biosensor for analysis of food ingredients. *European Food Research and Technology*, 235(3): 573-579.

Nakamura, H. (2018). Current status of water environment and their microbial biosensor techniques–Part II: Recent trends in microbial biosensor development. *Analytical and Bioanalytical Chemistry*, 410(17): 3967-3989.

Nicolopoulou-Stamati, P., Maipas, S., Kotampasi, C., Stamatis, P. & Hens, L. (2016). Chemical pesticides and human health: the urgent need for a new concept in agriculture. *Frontiers in Public Health*, 4: 148.

Pikkemaat, M. G., Rapallini, M. L., Karp, M. T. & Elferink, J. A. (2010). Application of a luminescent bacterial biosensor for the detection of tetracyclines in routine analysis of poultry muscle samples. *Food Additives and Contaminants*, 27(8): 1112-1117.

Raud, M., Linde, E., Kibena, E., Velling, S., Tenno, T., Talpsep, E. & Kikas, T. (2010). Semi□ specific biosensors for measuring BOD in dairy wastewater. *Journal of Chemical Technology & Biotechnology*, 85(7): 957-961.

Rotariu, L., Bala, C. & Magearu, V. (2002). Yeast cells sucrose biosensor based on a potentiometric oxygen electrode. *Analytica Chimica Acta*, 458(1): 215-222.

Rotariu, L., Bala, C. & Magearu, V. (2004). New potentiometric microbial biosensor for ethanol determination in alcoholic beverages. *Analytica Chimica Acta*, 513(1):119-123.

Sagiroglu, A., Paluzar, H., Ozcan, H.M., Okten, S. & Sen, B. (2011). A novel biosensor based on *Lactobacillus acidophilus* for determination of phenolic compounds in milk products and wastewater. *Preparative Biochemistry and Biotechnology*, 41(4): 321-336.

Scaria, J., Ramachandran, S., Jain, P. K. & Verma, S. K. (2009). Construction and testing of EGFP based bacterial biosensor for the detection of residual tetracyclines in milk and water. *Research Journal in Microbiology*, 4(3): 104-111.

Schenkmayerova, A., Bertokova, A., Sefcovicova, J., Stefuca, V., Bucko, M., Vikartovska, A., Gemeiner, P., Tkac, J. & Katrlík, J. (2015). Whole-cell *Gluconobacter oxydans* biosensor for 2-phenylethanol biooxidation monitoring. *Analytica Chimica Acta*, 854:140-144.

Sefcovicova, J., Filip. J. & Tkac. J. (2015). Interfacing of microbial cells with nanoparticles: simple and cost-effective preparation of a highly sensitive microbial ethanol biosensor. *Chemical Papers* 69: 176–82.

Sefcovicova, J., Filip. J., Mastihuba. V., Gemeiner. P. & Tkac. J. (2012). Analysis of ethanol in fermentation samples by a robust nanocomposite-based microbial biosensor. *Biotechnology Letters* 34(6): 1033-39.

Si, R. W., Yang. Y., Yu. Y. Y., et al. (2016). Wiring bacterial electron flow for sensitive whole-cell amperometric detection of riboflavin. *Analytical Chemistry* 88(22): 11222-28.

Stasyuk, N. Y., Gayda, G. Z. & Gonchar, M. V. (2014). l-Arginine-selective microbial amperometric sensor based on recombinant yeast cells over-producing human liver arginase I. *Sensors and Actuators B: Chemical*, 204: 515-521.

Tang, X., Zhang, T., Liang, B., Han, D., Zeng, L., Zheng, C., Li, T., Wei, M. & Liu, A. (2014). Sensitive electrochemical microbial biosensor for p-nitrophenylorganophosphates based on electrode modified with cell surface-displayed organophosphorus hydrolase and ordered mesopore carbons. *Biosensors and Bioelectronics*, 60: 137-142.

Valach, M., Katrlík, J., Sturdik, E. & Gemeiner, P. (2009). Ethanol *Gluconobacter* biosensor designed for flow injection analysis: Application in ethanol fermentation off-line monitoring. *Sensors and Actuators B: Chemical*, 138(2): 581-586.

Valimaa, A. L., Kivisto, A. T., Leskinen, P. I. & Karp, M. T. (2010). A novel biosensor for the detection of zearalenone family mycotoxins in milk. *Journal of Microbiological Methods*, 80(1): 44-48.

Verma, N. & Singh, M. (2003). A disposable microbial based biosensor for quality control in milk. *Biosensors and Bioelectronics*, 18(10): 1219-1224.

Verma, N. & Singh, M. (2006). A *Bacillus sphaericus* based biosensor for monitoring nickel ions in industrial effluents and foods. *Journal of Automated Methods and Management in Chemistry*, 1-4.

Verma, N., Kaur. H. & Kumar, S. (2011). Whole cell based electrochemical biosensor for monitoring lead ions in milk. *Biotechnology* 10(3): 259-66.

Verma, N., Kumar, S. & Kaur, H. (2011). Whole cell based disposable biosensor for Cadmium detection in milk. *Advances in Applied Science and Research* 2(6): 354-63.

Verma, N., Sharma, R. & Kumar, S. (2016). Advancement Towards Microfluidic Approach to Develop Economical Disposable Optical Biosensor for Lead Detection. *Austin Journal of Biosensors & Bioelectronics* 2(2): 1021.

Verma, N., Singh, A. K. & Singh, M. (2017). L-arginine biosensors: A comprehensive review. *Biochemistry and Biophysics Reports*, 12: 228-239.

Virolainen, N. E., Pikkemaat, M. G., Elferink, J. A. & Karp, M. T. (2008). Rapid detection of tetracyclines and their 4-epimer derivatives from poultry meat with bioluminescent biosensor bacteria. *Journal of Agricultural and Food Chemistry*, 56(23): 11065-11070.

Wen, G., Li, Z. & Choi, M. M. (2013). Detection of ethanol in food: A new biosensor based on bacteria. *Journal of Food Engineering*, 118(1): 56-61.

Wen, G., Wen, X., Shuang, S. & Choi, M. M. (2014). Whole-cell biosensor for determination of methanol. *Sensors and Actuators B: Chemical*, 201: 586-591.

Xu, X. & Ying, Y. (2011). Microbial biosensors for environmental monitoring and food analysis. *Food Reviews International*, *27*(3): 300-329.

Yu, Y. Y., Wang, J. X., Si, R. W., Yang, Y., Zhang, C. L. & Yong, Y. C. (2017). Sensitive amperometric detection of riboflavin with a whole-cell electrochemical sensor. *Analytica Chimica Acta,* 985: 148-54.

Yue, H., He, Y., Fan, E., Wang, L., Lu, S. & Fu, Z. (2017). Label-free electrochemiluminescent biosensor for rapid and sensitive detection of *pseudomonas aeruginosa* using phage as highly specific recognition agent. *Biosensors and Bioelectronics,* 94: 429-32.

Zhang, Z., Liu, J., Fan, J., Wang, Z. & Li, L. (2018). Detection of catechol using an electrochemical biosensor based on engineered *Escherichia coli* cells that surface-display laccase. *Analytica Chimica Acta*, 1009: 65-72.

7

Fourier Transform Infrared (FTIR) Spectroscopy: Principle and Application in Analysis of Dairy Products

Akshay Ramani[1], Chandrakanta Sen[1], Pavel Rout[1] and Shamim Hossain[2*]

[1]Dairy Chemistry Division, ICAR-National Dairy Research Institute, Karnal Haryana
[2]Dairy Technology Division, ICAR-National Dairy Research Institute Karnal, Haryana

Abstract

Fourier transform infrared (FTIR) spectroscopy is called a "fingerprint" technique because no two different samples are known to give the same spectrum. It can be used for solid, liquid, or gaseous samples, which give spectra based on the vibrational transitions happening in the molecule. This chapter focuses on how FTIR spectroscopy can be used to improve food quality and safety. This is done to make it easier for young, creative food technologists to understand and build their knowledge.

Introduction

Fourier transform infrared (FTIR) spectroscopy is one of the most effective methods for determining the functional groups and potential molecular interactions between membrane chemical molecules. Understanding of (infrared) IR absorption band placements in the spectrum as wave numbers can be used to identify the various chemical constituents (such as aromatic amides) that may not be visible by X-ray photoelectron spectroscopy. In general, IR spectroscopy is applicable to a wide range of substances. It could be applied for qualitative and quantitative study of materials and condition. Recently, the attenuated total reflectance (ATR) method has gained more interest for characterization due to its access to surface vibrational frequencies bulk substance.

The majority of the first portion of this book chapter is describing FTIR Principle and vibrational spectroscopy, while the second section is devoted to describing sample analysis, applications of FTIR spectroscopy in dairy products. The fundamental principle of sample handling techniques for FTIR spectroscopy includes the following: Absorption of transmission, ATR, diffuse reflection, and true specular reflectance/reflection. This section of the chapter will describe the application of FTIR spectroscopy. Monitoring the surface functionalization of membranes utilising a variety of techniques. In addition, this chapter provides an overview of the application of FTIR spectroscopy for stability analysis and durability of membrane in a variety of applications, including gas separation of water and fuel cells. Utilizing FTIR spectroscopy to identify the chemical composition by distinguishing a range of functional groups, components explain or emphasise their function in membrane functionality.

Vibrational Spectroscopy

The chemical, petrochemical, polymer, pharmaceutical, cosmetic, culinary, and agricultural industries' growing need to improve product quality and rationalise production has significantly revived the vibrational spectroscopic field. Spectroscopic methods utilising Raman, IR, and (Near infrared) NIR technology have contributed to the gradual replacement of conservative analytical methods that take a lot of time such as high-performance liquid chromatography and gas chromatography (HPLC), Mass spectrometry (MS), nuclear magnetic resonance (NMR), and non-specific control techniques (temperature, pressure, pH, dosing weights). Vibrational spectroscopy is a highly specialised and ecologically friendly analytical technique.

Classical Model

The molecules are thought to act like harmonic oscillators in the classical model. A harmonic oscillator is a system in which a mass is coupled to a spring with a set spring constant (B). A restoring force begins acting on a particle of mass "m" when we move it out of its equilibrium position, attempting to return it to its original location. If the particle is displaced along the x-axis, the restoring force acting on it is given by the formula:

$$F = -kx \tag{1}$$

Where, F is the restoring force, k is the spring constant, and x is the length of the spring's extension along the x-axis.

The rate of change of momentum can be calculated using Newton's second law as follows:

$F = ma = md^2x/dt^2$ (2)

Thus what we get from Eqns. (1) and (2) is

$d^2x/dt^2+\omega^2x = 0$ dt,

a second-order linear differential equation with an oscillatory solution, is.

$x = A\sin \omega t$ (3),

where; $\omega = \sqrt{k/m}$ is the frequency of vibration, k is spring constant and m mass of single-particle.

A system of two particles coupled to a spring with a spring constant of k. Using the equations above, we can determine the frequency of vibration for this system, which is represented by Eqn (4).

$\omega = \sqrt{k/\mu}$ (4)

Where; $\mu = m_1m_2/m_1+m_2$ = is reduced mass of system.

Similar to this, in order to forecast how a particle would behave in a system of more than two particles, we must solve differential equations in more complicated situations. However, in a two-particle system, there are two distinct vibrational modes that can either be in phase or out of phase. According to the conventional model, the system oscillates continuously with energy.

Traditionally, kinetic and potential energy are added to create total energy, as seen below:

$E = T + V$ (5)

When T and V, respectively, are kinetic and potential energies, are expressed as follows:

$T = 1/2m\ (dx/dt)^2$ (6)

$V=1/2\ kx^2$ (7)

At the oscillator's equilibrium position, the potential energy is zero and the oscillator's total energy is solely kinetic; at the turning point, the potential energy is zero and the oscillator's total energy is solely potential. While the quantum mechanical model, according to the Planck harmonic oscillator, has the discrete form of energy, the classical model's oscillator can have a continuous value of energy.

Quantum Mechanical Analysis

German physicist Max Planck proposed in 1900 that the oscillator in the cavity has discrete values of energy rather than a continuous value of energy. He claims that when two energy levels (E^1 and E^2) transition, the energy changes and is stated as follows:

$$\Delta E = E_2 - E_1 = hv \tag{8}$$

Where, v is the frequency of the radiation and h is the Planck's constant.

When electromagnetic (EM) radiations interact with molecules, the radiation is absorbed by the molecule and an energy state shift between E_1 and E_2 takes place. Because there are several energy levels that correspond to potential transitions, the spectra of molecules are becoming more complex. Vibrational spectroscopy, in which molecules interact with EM radiation and begin vibrating with various modes of vibration and these modes have discrete values of energy, analyses the simple and complicated spectra of molecules.

Vibrational Spectrum

This section discusses how electromagnetic radiation affects molecular vibration. The Schrodinger equation can be solved to determine the energy, wavenumber, and potential frequency mode of vibrating molecules. When a molecule interacts with an electromagnetic wave, it has vibrational energy. Let's assume the most basic scenario for a diatomic molecule's vibration, which is comparable to the vibration of a spring attached with two masses, m_1 and m_2, to analyse the spectroscopy of a molecule (B). Such a system's Schrodinger equation is:

$$\nabla^2 + 8^2\mu/h^2 \times (E-V) = 0 \tag{9}$$

Where, m is the reduced mass, E is the system's total energy, and V is the potential energy ($V = \frac{1}{2}kx^2$), is a wave function that provides all the information about the system that is required.

Similar to a spring, a bond's compression or extension abides by Hook's law. There are three dimensions in equation (9). The spring's extension or compression is in one dimension, hence the equation (9) in one dimension can be represented as follows:

$$d^2\frac{\varphi}{dx^2} + \frac{8\pi^2\mu}{h^2}\left(E - \frac{1}{2}kx^2\right)\varphi = 0 \tag{10}$$

To determine the energy of a vibrating molecule, we solve Eqn. (10) and get at:

$$E_v = \frac{h}{2\pi}\frac{\sqrt{k}}{\mu}\left(v+\frac{1}{2}\right) = hv_{osc}\left(v+\frac{1}{2}\right), v = 0,1,2,3,..... \qquad (11)$$

In wavenumber representation, we have Eqn. (12):

$$\varepsilon_v = \frac{E_v}{hc} = {}^{v_{osc}}\!/_{c}\left(v+\frac{1}{2}\right) = \frac{\omega}{2\pi c}\left(v+\frac{1}{2}\right) = \omega_e\left(v+\frac{1}{2}\right) \qquad (12)$$

Subsequently for each vibrational quantum number, we get:

$$\varepsilon_v = \frac{1}{2}\omega_e, \frac{3}{2}\omega_e, \frac{5}{2}\omega_e, ...v = 0,1,2...... \qquad (13)$$

Where, v is a vibrational quantum number.

This shows that the vibrational levels are distinct, evenly spaced, and have a common spacing of cm^{-1}. In terms of wavenumber, we have discovered the energy of a vibrating oscillator. This quantized energy value of the vibrating molecules is calculated under the assumption that the molecules are moving in a simple harmonic motion and that the potential profile corresponding to this motion is precisely parabolic. However, because the bonds between molecules in actuality are not as homogenous as they are in the case of a spring-mass system, molecules do not adhere to harmonic oscillation and Hook's law. As a result, we must take into account a brand-new potential profile that includes the total molecular signature. This potential profile is called a harmonic potential, and the oscillator that corresponds to it is called a harmonic oscillator.

Anharmonic oscillator's potential is:

$$v(r) = f(r-r^e)^2 - g(r - r^e)^3 = fx^2 - gx^3 \qquad (14)$$

The energy values of Anharmonic oscillator is:

$$\varepsilon_v = hc\omega_e\left(v+\frac{1}{2}\right) - hc\omega_e x_e\left(v+\frac{1}{2}\right)^2 \qquad (15)$$

Where, is the anharmonic constant, and ω is the spacing between energy levels when the potential energy curve is a parabola. The value of " $\omega_e x_e < x_e$ " shows that the energy levels of the anharmonic oscillator are not equally spaced out.

The selection rule is a set of guidelines that governs the transition between any two vibrational energy levels. The following are the selection criteria (Eqn. (16)): $\Delta v = \pm 1, \pm 2, \pm 3, ...$

This is the general discussion about the interaction of EM radiations with the vibrating diatomic molecules, which can be applied to several other molecules. As a food technologist, we want to employ this concept to food, which is a complex system involving several molecules and their bonds, for example, amide in proteins, carboxyl in lipids, etc. Therefore, transition between the energy levels of these molecules is also governed by the said selection rule and are exploited for several purposes that will be discussed in the latter part of this chapter.

Working Principles

FTIR is an analytical instrument which is used to study the interaction of infrared light with the matter. The output of an FTIR is a plot of measured infrared radiation intensity versus wavenumber (called an infrared spectrum). The instrument that determines the absorption spectrum for a compound is called a spectrophotometer. When compared to a conventional spectrophotometer, a Fourier transform spectrophotometer provides the IR spectrum much more quickly. The major part of a basic FTIR spectrophotometer is schematically shown in figure 7.1. The device generates an IR beam that is emanated from a luminous black-body source. The interferometer is a component where the spectral encoding originates after the beam enters it. An interferogram, also known as constructive and destructive interference, is produced by the recombination of beams with various path lengths in the interferometer. The beam now enters the sample compartment, where it is absorbed by the sample at precise frequencies that are specific to the sample from the interferogram. The detector then simultaneously measures the energy against time for all frequencies of the particular interferogram signal. A beam is superimposed in the interim to serve as a reference (background) for the instrument's operation. After the interferogram automatically eliminated the background spectrum from the sample spectrum using Fourier transformation computer software, the desired spectrum was finally obtained.

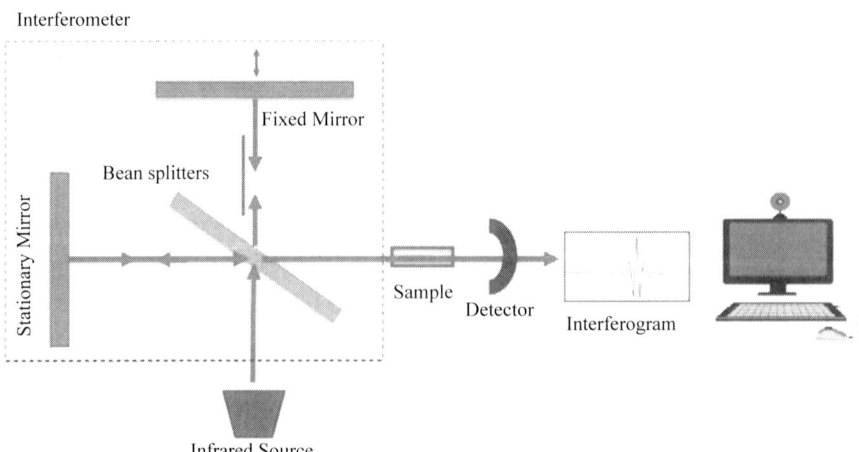

Fig. 7.1: Schematic Diagram of FTIR Components

Basically, the mid-IR area 2.5-15 mm between 4000 and 666 cm^{-1} is where the IR spectrum from the FTIR spectrometer is located. The appearance of an absorption band in the mid-IR region (4000-400 cm^{-1}) can be used to ascertain whether specific functional groups are present in the molecule because transition energies corresponding to changes in vibrational energy state for many functional groups are located there (4000-400 cm^{-1}). Generally, the FTIR spectra can be used to investigate four zones of different bond types. Figure 7.2 illustrates that single bonds (O-H, C-H, and N-H) can be detected in higher wavenumbers (2500-4000 cm^{-1}). Furthermore, the middle wavenumber regions of 2000-2500 cm^{-1} and 1500-2000 cm^{-1} respectively allow for the detection of the triple bond and the double bond. A complex pattern of vibrations at low wavenumber area 650-1500 cm^{-1} that are characteristic of the molecule as a whole and can be utilised for identification are also produced by the vibration of the molecule as a whole. For instance, the FTIR measurement of the regenerated cellulose membranes in Fig 2 showed the distinctive cellulose signal. C-O-C stretching at cellulose's b-linked glucose is something that is responsible for the band at 891 cm^{-1}. Additionally, the C-O-C pyranose ring's stretching vibration (see inset image) produced a shoulder band at 1053 cm^{-1}, which corresponds to the amount of cellulose in the regenerated cellulose membrane (RCM).

In short, the IR spectrum is divided into three wavenumber regions: the far-IR spectrum (400 cm^{-1}), the mid-IR spectrum (400–4000 cm^{-1}), and the near-IR spectrum (4000-13000 cm^{-1}). Most of the time, the mid-IR spectrum is used to analyse samples, but the far-IR and near-IR spectrum can also give information about the samples being looked at. This study was mostly about analysing FTIR in the mid-IR range.

The mid-IR spectrum is split into four parts:

a) single bond region (2500–4000 cm^{-1}),

b) double bond region (1500–2000 cm^{-1}),

c) triple bond region (2000–2500 cm^{-1}),

d) fingerprint region (600-1500 cm^{-1}).

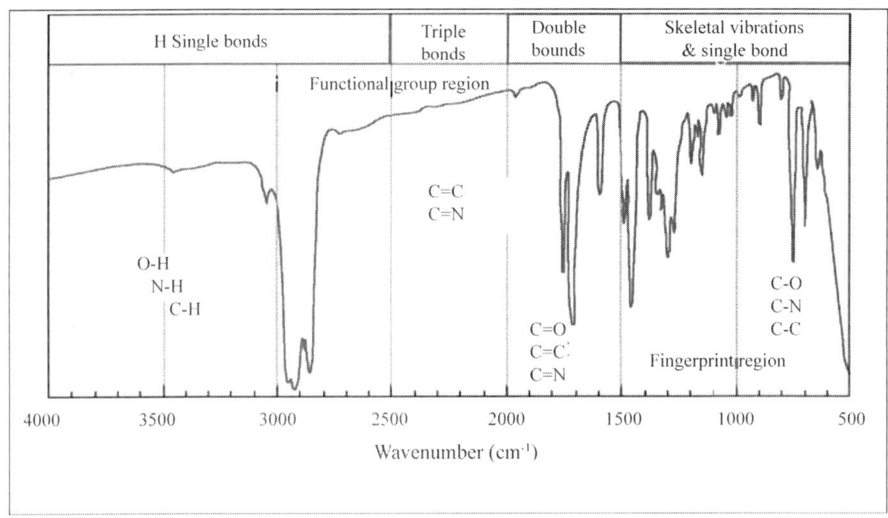

Fig. 7.2: FTIR spectrum

FTIR components

The components of the FTIR spectrophotometer are described in brief in the below paragraph. The different components play different functions and connected to each other in the specific sequence.

The Source

Infrared radiation is typically generated by an electrically conducting filament, the specific of which depend on the wavelength range of IR being investigated. Typically, silicon carbide Nernst filaments and Globar filaments are used in the MIR range.

Interferometer

One of the most popular interferometers used in FTIR is the Michelson interferometer. This is comprised of a beam splitter, a moving mirror, and a fixed mirror (Figure 7.3) from the source to the interferometer, a parallel beam of radiation is transmitted and initially reaches the beam splitter. The beam splitter is a semi-reflective transparent film that divides the beam into two halves that each contain 50% of the radiation. The amount of radiation in each split beam and the resulting IR spectral region are dependent on the construction material of the beam splitter. Typically, germanium or iron oxide-coated potassium bromide or caesium iodide substrates are used for the MIR region. As the radiation beam is split at the bisecting plane in front of the two aluminized or silver-surfaced mirrors, one of the split beams is reflected at

90° to the stationary mirror, while the other half is allowed to pass directly towards the moving mirror. The moving mirror is constantly aligned with a visible helium-neon (He-Ne) laser that is focused at the mirror's corner in order to ensure accurate distance scanning and more precise measurements. Once the two radiation beams have been reflected by the two mirrors, they are recombined at the beam splitter and directed at 90° to the source and towards the sample as a single transmitted beam. Since each beam travels a different distance due to the relative position changes between the moving and stationary mirrors, an interference pattern is created where the beams converge. Depending on the distance travelled by the second beam, the radiation waves can either recombine in phase, interfering constructively, or out of phase, interfering destructively. Thus, IR radiation at all wavelengths is attained. Once the transmitted beam has been formed, it will pass through the sample, where a portion of its energy will be absorbed. The remaining portion reaches the detector, where the interferogram is recorded and then translated using Fourier transformation into the sample absorbance spectrum.

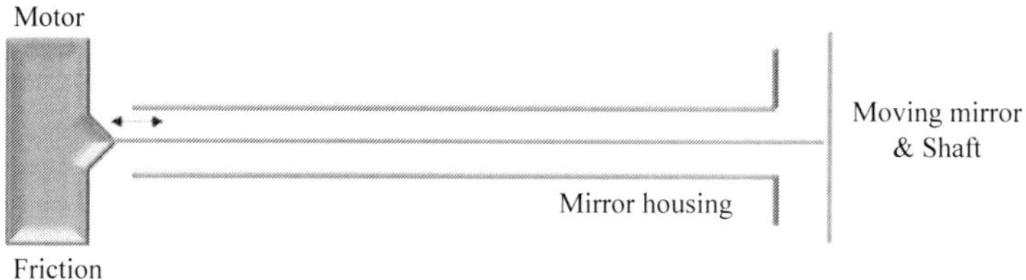

Fig. 7.3: The illustration how the Interferometer works in a FTIR

The Sample

The beam enters the sample compartment, where, depending on the type of analysis being performed, it is either transmitted through or reflected by the sample's surface. At this point, certain frequencies of energy, which are exclusive to the sample, are absorbed. These frequencies are uniquely characterised by the sample.

Beam-splitter

The beam-splitter is the most important part of the interferometer, as shown in Figure 7.1 Remember that the beam-splitter's job is to take an infrared beam, split it in two, and then put the two beams back together into one. The way a beam-splitter works is shown in Figure 7.4. Most FTIRs have a thin film of germanium between two windows that let infrared light pass through. This is called a beam splitter. The thickness of the germanium is just right for some infrared radiation to pass through and some to rebound.

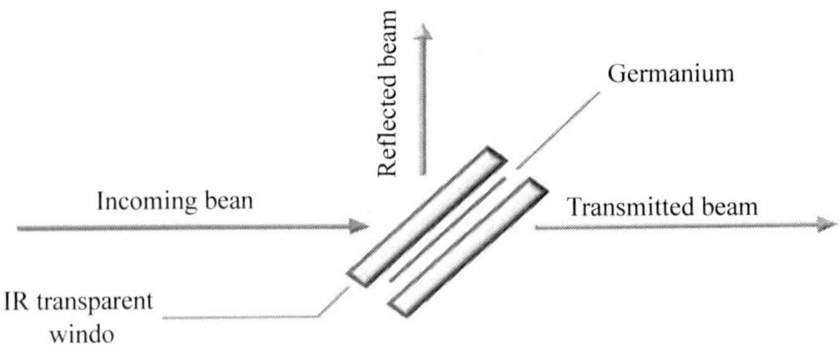

Fig. 7.4: The illustration how the beam splitter works in a FTIR

It's like a two-way mirror with a thin layer of silver that can reflect and transmit light. A glass pane can split light. You can see through a pane of glass, which indicates it transmits visible light, but you can also see your reflection, which means it reflects visible light. Beam-splitter infrared windows support and protect germanium film. FTIRs have KBr beam-splitters. KBr is transparent from 400 cm^{-1} to the near-infrared and easy to manufacture. Many FTIRs contain beam-splitters with KBr windows. KBr is useful because it is clear over a wide range of wavelengths, from 400 cm^{-1} to the near-infrared, and is easy to work. Most FTIR can't measure spectra below 400 cm^{-1} because at that point, the KBr windows in the beam-splitter start to absorb light very strongly. One of the most common drawback of the KBr is that it absorbs water from the air because it is hygroscopic.

Detectors

IR detectors are also different depending on the IR range being studied. There are two primary types of detectors: thermocouple detectors, which measure the heating effect of radiation, and photoconductor detectors, which measure the conductivity produced by IR radiation. The deuteratedtriglycinesulphate (DTGS) pyroelectric detector is a common detector for the MIR region. It is usually placed in an alkali halide window, which is resistant to heat, and the mercury cadmium telluride (MCT) photoconductive detectors need to be cooled to liquid nitrogen temperatures, but they are more sensitive and respond faster.

The Computer

The measured signal is converted to digital form and sent to the computer, where the Fourier transformation. The user is then shown the final infrared spectrum for interpretation and any additional manipulation.

Sampling Techniques

FTIR uses the entire source range, in which all wavelengths are recorded simultaneously as opposed to covering the individual wavelengths produced by the grating and prism system used in dispersive spectroscopy, and multiple scans can be averaged in the same time as a single spectrum is taken with a dispersive spectrometer (Stuart, 2000). For testing with complicated structures, such as food matrices, reflectance approaches have been chosen as an alternative to the most seasoned and clear transmission strategies. In reflectance, the beam reflected back from the sample is measured, and based on the kind of reflectance, either from a cell in contact with the sample or directly from the sample, reflectance measurements can be classed as internal or external (Stuart, 2000; 2004).

Diffuse Reflectance

External reflectance estimates surface radiation. In DRS, infrared light is directed on a sample cup containing KBr-mixed sample, and the reflected light is captured by a mirror and measured by a detector. Particle size affects spectral intensity (Stuart, 2004). Jaiswal and co-workers estimated banana quality (Jaiswal *et al.,* 2015) and mango sweetness (Jha *et al.,* 2015) using diffuse reflectance sampling. The authors gathered spectra at 299–1100 nm for 95 bananas using a portable NIR spectrometer and applied regression models, partial least square, and multilinear regression algorithms on complete range of spectral data (Jaiswal *et al.,* 2015; Jha *et al.,* 2015).

Photoacoustic Spectroscopy (PAS)

Photoacoustic spectroscopy (PAS) is based on how tweaked infrared radiation is changed into mechanical vibration. In this method, the sample is placed on a sample cup that has helium or air in it. Modulated infrared radiation warms and cools a sample when absorbed. Helium absorbs heat, expands, and creates pressure waves. A microphone converts pressure waves to electronic signals. The background is carbon black. This non-invasive technology works for all samples. PAS is beneficial since the measured signal is proportional to the sample concentration (Silverstein *et al.,* 2014; Stuart *et al.,* 2004). FTIR-PAS uses a portable, variable-speed mirror for depth profiling in many fields. Lv *et al.* (2018) detected fungicide in rice using FTIR-PAS. Liu *et al.* (2015) used PAS and ANN (artificial neural network) to quantify dichlorvos residues on apple cuticle.

Attenuated Total Reflectance (ATR)

ATR is popular due to its fast response. It can examine materials of varying morphology or physical state. In this procedure, infrared beam is completely reflected when it hits a sample. Thus, the thickness of the absorbing samples is not important, as it is in transmission radiation, as long as full surface contact is provided. ATR uses total internal reflectance, which occurs when radiation travels through two media at an angle larger than the critical angle (Granato *et al.,* 2018). In ATR accessories, infrared radiation is reflected through optically thick crystal while interacting with the sample, and absorbance information is acquired.

It's an adaptable method for easy infrared examination and useful for examining smooth materials that are too thick or foggy for transmission estimates. ATR is non-destructive, requiring almost no sample preparation, and allows quick and easy food testing (fluid, gel, powder, etc.). To collect high-quality spectral data, sample and crystal must have great contact (Justice *et al.,* 1999).

Specular Reflectance

Two mirrors are utilized for specular reflectance. One mirror sends the light onto the sample, while another mirror directs the reflected IR beam to the detector. The history is gathered against a gold reflected surface. It requires a smooth sample surface and has been effectively utilized in polymer research (Justice *et al.,* 1999; Stuart *et al.,* 2004). Powdered samples are suitable for specular reflection measurements, despite the requirement that the sample surface must be smooth, necessitating the use of a surface coating in certain applications of Chemometric Fourier Transform Infrared (FTIR) Spectroscopy.

Chemometrics

Chemometrics (sometimes called chemoinformatics) extracts information about chemical systems using mathematics, statistics, and computer science. Analyzed data allows for optimal measurement processes and tests, yielding maximal chemical information (Haghiri, 2016). It covers chemistry, biology, medicine, biochemistry, and chemical engineering.

Rapid technical advances have permitted the production of high-dimensional (HD) data in many fields. HD data has hundreds, thousands, or millions of dimensions, such as absorbance/transmittance in FTIR spectral data. Since our brain only works in three dimensions, it's tough to understand multidimensional data display. Data dimensionality must be reduced or simplified. This can be done by grouping related data using multidimensional scaling to discover similarities or clustering in-group data. FTIR delivers data at useful and uninformative regions for a specific analyte; analysing the complete region won't disclose significant information. Before data analysis, the undesired regions/signals/noise from HD data are removed/reduced by selecting the required wavenumber range, data pre-processing (DP), or data pre-treatment (DPT). Unsupervised (used often owing to efficiency and simplicity) and supervised DP algorithms exist. Unsupervised approach can be column- or row-wise. The dataset is transformed column-wise by centering and scaling. Minor changes in dataset composition affect the converted data matrix. Row-wise operations change each spectrum separately. Thus, dataset composition changes don't effect processed data. Orthogonal signal correction (OSC) is an example of reference-dependent approaches (supervised data) (Bureau *et al.*, 2009; Sun, 2009). Discrete wavelet transforms and wavelet packet transform.

Standard Normal Variate (SNV)

This normalisation method corrects changes in global signal intensity caused by light scattering, radiation penetration, or sample size. SNV has mean μ=0 and standard deviation (σ)=1. Interaction of IR radiations with sample particle often results in a change of absorbance levels as light scattering produces differences in route length and background signal levels with wavelength. Baseline shift and curvature result. This can vary between samples and complicate spectral interpretation and linear calibration of NIR diffuse reflectance spectra. Barnes *et al.* (1993) devised SNV modification to reduce scattering and particle size multiplicative effects and signal intensity differences. This enhances PLS model prediction for NIR scattering data. SNV assumes multiplicative effects are homogeneous across the spectral range, which can lead to artefacts (which is not true always). First, each spectrum is centred, then scaled by (Ye, 2007).

Multiplicative Scatter Correction

It corrects additive (like path length disparities) and multiplicative (like particle size) scattering effects, which are not due to the sample's chemical make-up but to its measurement geometry and morphology. Before performing MSC, two assumptions are made: first, the sample spectrum is a result of adding two spectra, i.e., absorption by chemical bonds (which we want to retain) and diffusion/scattering of light (which we want to reduce); second, all samples show the same coefficient of diffusion spectrum at all wavelengths, which can be modelled via least-squares using a reference spectrum. MSC requires a reference spectrum, which SNV lacks. From (a) and (b), it's evident that each spectrum's structure can be owing to three factors: (a) absorption of different wavelengths of IR radiations by the sample, leading to a specific spectrum due to the chemical nature of sample and of our interest; (b) difference in particle size of sample which causes radiations to deviate at a different angle as per the wavelength (i.e., scattering effect); (c) difference in path length arising due to variation in sample position and/or surface irregularities, leading to variations in sp. SNV and MSC reduce (1) and (2). Outliers require SNV.

Principal Component Analysis (PCA)

It's a descriptive statistical tool and adaptive exploratory strategy used to reduce the HD dataset's dimensionality while preserving its variability (a reservoir of statistical information).

Multivariate data analysis uses PCA. Principal components (PC) are linear functions of the original dataset. The first PC has the largest variance among all linear combinations (Downey *et al.,* 1997). PCA is also helpful in linear regression and simultaneous individual and variable clustering (in the form of biplots). Incremental PCA (IPCA), sparse PCA (sPCA), etc. have been adapted for data analysis. Low-rank approximation is built into IPCA when the dataset is large enough to fit in memory. sPCA is a PCA-based model with sparse scores and/or loadings. sPCA loses PC non-correlation and loading vector orthogonality (Settle, 1997). Camacho *et al.* (2019) compares sPCA and PCA's advantages, weaknesses, and assumptions.

Partial Least Square (PLS)

It is a statistical strategy for projecting the future that combines PCA with multiple regressions. It is used to predict a set of dependent variables from a large collection of independent variables by calculating the regression coefficient in a linear model containing a large number of strongly correlated x-variables. During calibration, this technique uses information from both matrices, i.e., spectroscopic data (X) and concentration (Y), and compresses data to account for the majority of variations caused by X and Y. Consequently, the potential impact of fluctuations in X during calibration is diminished (Araujo *et al.,* 2001).

Successive Projection Algorithm (SPA)

It is a forward variable selection approach suggested by Araujo *et al.* (2001). In MLR (multiple linear regression, which uses explanatory variables for predicting outcome of response variable by explaining the relationship between a single continuous dependent variable and >1 independent variable which may be continuous or discrete), wavelengths containing minimally redundant information are chosen to minimise co-linearity problems (which refers to the situation in which some independent variables are highly correlated). In multiple applications of NIR spectroscopy, SPA-MLR is reportedly more accurate in predicting outcomes than PLS/PCR models (Ye, 2007).

Linear Discriminant Analysis (LDA)

It is a supervised algorithm model for achieving maximal class reparability of data by lowering data dimensionality and classifying HD data into low-dimensional space.

Self Organizing Maps (SOM)

Kohonen maps, also known as SOM maps, were developed by Teuvo Kohonen (1995). Comparable to the score plot of principal component analysis, this method employs a non-linear approach to depicting HD data in a 2-dimensional plot (map). Since PCA is a linear projection approach, SOM should be used if it does not work. The primary goal of SOM is cluster analysis (i.e., exploratory data analysis). In this map depicts the Squares close to one other contain objects with comparable descriptions.

Cross Validation (CV) and Bootstrap

Both are internal validation techniques for separating data into calibration and test sets. Model construction and optimization employ calibration/training set. The test set is then tested on the calibration set model to forecast performance realistically. CV or bootstrap are resampling algorithms for tiny data sets. Bootstrapping with replacements is better than a single CV.

Sampling Algorithm and Random Algorithm

Both are external validation methods, but internal validation solely considers sample variability (Justice *et al.,* 1999). In our scenario, suppose we first capture spectra, apply required chemometric procedures, and then create an internal validation model by testing known samples (milk) for an analyte (some antibiotic) (Geanato *et al.,* 2018). For verifying this model's efficiency, we can obtain milk samples from various producers (making these independent sets of samples) and run the algorithm to see if it works in field space.

The root mean square error of calibration and the root mean square error of prediction (RMSEP), as well as residuals and the selection of the calibration variable factor, are highly essential factors to take into consideration and have importance in the NIR method in terms of accuracy and precision.

FTIR Data Analysis

Spectrum in the FTIR analysis

The main point of the FTIR analysis is to figure out what the FTIR spectrum means (see example FTIR spectrum in Figure 7.2). Data about "absorption versus wavenumber" or "transmission versus wavenumber" can be found in the spectrum.

FTIR analysis aims to interpret the spectrum. The spectrum contains absorption and transmission data. Far-IR (400 cm^{-1}), mid-IR (400–4000 cm^{-1}), and near-IR are the three IR wavenumber ranges (4000-13000 cm^{-1}). Mid-IR is usually utilised to assess samples, but far-IR and near-IR can also provide information.

Step 1: Determine the total number of absorption band

- Determine the total number of absorption bands that are present in the IR spectra. If the spectrum of the sample is straightforward (has less than five absorption bands), then the molecules being analysed are either simple organic compounds, compounds with a low molecular weight, or inorganic compounds (such as simple salts). However, if the FTIR spectrum shows more than 5 different absorption bands, the substance under investigation may be a complex compound.

Step 2: Determining single bond region (2500-4000 cm^{-1}). There are a number of peaks in this region

- A 3650-3250 cm^{-1} absorption band indicating a hydrogen bond. This band signifies H_2O, hydroxyl, or amino. Followed by hydroxyl spectra at 1600–1300, 1200–1000, and 800–600 cm^{-1}. Sharp absorption at 3670 and 3550 cm^{-1} suggests the chemical contains an oxygen-related group, like an alcohol or phenol (illustrates the absence of hydrogen bonding).

- 3000 cm^{-1} narrow band indicating unsaturated compounds or aromatic rings. Simple unsaturated olefinic molecules absorb between 3010 and 3040 cm^{-1}.

- Narrow band below 3000 cm^{-1} indicating aliphatic compounds. Linear aliphatic compounds with long chain lengths absorb at 2935 and 2860 cm^{-1}. Peaks between 1470 and 720 cm^{-1} follow the bond.

- The specific aldehyde peak is located between 2700 and 2800 cm^{-1}.

Step 3: Identifying the region of triple bonds (2000-2500 cm^{-1})

- A peak at 2200 cm^{-1} may be C's absorption band. The peak usually appears after additional spectra at 1600-1300, 1200-1000, and 800-600 cm^{-1}.

Step 4: Identifying the double bond region (1500-2000 cm^{-1})

Carbonyl (C = C), amino (C = N), and azo (N = N) groups can form double bonds.

- For carbonyl compounds, 1850 to 1650 cm^{-1}
- Above 1775 cm^{-1}, anhydrides, halide acids, halogenated carbonyl, or ring-carbonyl carbons such lactone or organic carbonate.
- In range1750-1700 cm^{-1}, simple carbonyl compounds like ketones, aldehydes, esters, and carboxyl.
- Amides or carboxylates respond below 1700 cm^{-1}.
- If a carbonyl group is conjugated with another, double-bond and aromatic peak intensities are reduced. Aldehydes, ketones, esters, and carboxylic acids inhibit carbonyl absorption.
- 1670-1620 cm^{-1} for unsaturated bond (double and triple bond). Double-bond carbon or olefinic compounds (C = C) peak at 1650 cm^{-1}. Normal conjugations with C = C, C = O, or aromatic rings reduce the frequency of intense absorption bands. Unsaturated bond diagnosis requires absorption below 3000 cm^{-1}. C-H absorbs between 3085 and 3025 cm. C-H absorbs over 3000 cm^{-1}.
- A strong intensity between 1650 and 1600 cm^{-1}, which informs double bonds or aromatic substances.
- Response aromatic ring between 1615-1495 cm^{-1}, between 1600 and 1500 cm^{-1}, two absorption bands formed. These aromatic rings have mild to moderate absorption between 3150 and 3000 cm^{-1} (for C-H stretching).

Step 5: Identifying the fingerprint region (600-1500 cm^{-1})

This area is typically specific and unique.

- Within a wavelength range of 1000 to 880 cm^{-1}, there are absorption bands located at 1650, 3010 and 3040 cm^{-1}. These bands are used for multiple band absorption.

- It should be paired with absorption bands at 1650, 3010, and 3040 cm^{-1}, all of which display characteristics of compound unsaturation, in order to achieve the C-H transition (out-of-plane bending).
- When discussing compounds that are related to vinyl, the frequency range of approximately 900 to 990 cm^{-1} is used to identify vinyl terminals ($-CH=CH_2$), the frequency range of 965 to 960 cm^{-1} is used to identify trans unsaturated vinyl (CH=CH), and the frequency range of 890 cm^{-1} is used to identify double olefinic bonds in single vinyl ($C=CH_2$).
- When it comes to aromatic compounds, a single, robust absorption band may be detected in the range of 750 cm^{-1} for orto and 830 cm^{-1} for para. Both of these regions correspond to the same wavelength.

Application in Dairy Product Analysis

Food is a nutrient-rich solid or liquid that, when eaten, is digested and used by the body to keep it healthy and fit. The parts of food can be categorised into proteins, carbohydrates, fat, vitamins, minerals, and water-based not only on what they do in the body, but also on the fact that the majority of chemical bonds (except for minerals) are found in these classes, such as:

Table 7.1: Chemical bonds mainly present in dairy products

Fats	C–H; C = O; C = C – H
Proteins	Amide I, C=O; Amide II, N–H, C–N
Carbohydrates	C–H; C–O
Water	O–H; H–O–H
Alcohol	O–H; C–O
Amine	N-H; C-N; N-H
Aromatic	C-H; C=C
Carbonyl	C=O
Ether	C–O

From what we've talked about so far, it's clear that FTIR works on the vibrational changes that happen in molecules, which are unique to each molecule. So, these vibrational changes happen at a certain wavenumber for a certain molecule or bond. Since food is a complicated thing with both large and small molecules that can absorb IR radiation, the spectra that are made for food are harder to understand. Because of this, using chemometrics in food matrices is even more useful. But it is very interesting to note that the spectra of no two different foods overlap. This makes FTIR a fingerprinting method.

FTIR can be used in food systems to find out what the food is made of and to learn about the properties of the macronutrients it contains (Silverstein *et al.,* 2014). When FTIR is combined with chemometrics, it can be used in food science and related fields, such as microbiology, the effect of processing, monitoring oxidation processes in oil, etc. to get qualitative and/or quantitative information about the food. It has been used a lot to study the quality and safety of foods, which is what this chapter is about.

Quality is usually defined as how well something is done. Quality of food refers to a set of things about a product, like its taste, texture, colour, nutritive value, fat content, etc., that all work together to make a consumer decide whether or not to buy it. On the other hand, food safety focuses on keeping food from having any chemical or biological toxins or potential toxins, or too much of a food additive (Hacisalihoglu *et al.,* 2010).

Dairy Industry

Dairy industry is booming all over the world, and FTIR has been used a lot to figure out what is in milk. In addition, it is frequently used to determine the safety and quality of milk.

Coitinho *et al.* (2017) used FTIR to keep an eye on things like corn-starch, sodium bicarbonate, formaldehyde, sodium citrate, and saccharose that were added to milk, as well as the addition of water or whey. The researchers did the analysis with the FTIR MilkoScan FT1 instrument, which scans the whole middle infrared region from 2.0 to 10.8 m (5012 to 926 cm^{-1}) in wavelengths. Leite *et al.* (2019) used the ATR-FTIR and PCA models to find soybean oil, which is now being used to replace butter oil in the preparation of butter cheese as an adulterant. The authors said that a band at 3007.1 cm^{-1} appeared as the amount of soybean oil used to replace butter oil went up.

Table 7.2: Applications of FTIR spectroscopy in quality milk and dairy products

Applications Significant	Chemometric technique used	Wavelength Used	Results	References
Detection of beef fat in butter	PCR, PLS	3873-690 cm^{-1}	The lowest amount of palm oil that can be detection in butter is 3%, and the lowest amount that can be measured is 9.8%.	Ranvir *et al.*, 2018
Cholesterol Estimation in Dairy Products	PCR, PLS	2800 and 3200 cm^{-1}	Results indicate that FTIR spectroscopy can determine the cholesterol content in dairy products in approximately 5 min.	Paradkar *et al.*, 2002
Detection of the microbial spoilage in milk	Multivariate statistical method, including PCA, PLS	4000-600 cm^{-1}	Results were good for bacterial loads over 105 cfu/ml.	Nicolaou & Goodacre, 2008
Detection of species adulteration of milk	PLS regression and nonlinear kernel partial least squares regressions	4000 to 600 cm^{-1}	When combined with multivariate analysis like linearPLS and nonlinear Kernel PLS, FT-IR spectroscopy is a quick, easy, and accurate way to figure out how much sheep, goat, and cow milk has been adulterated.	Nicolaou *et al.*, 2010
FTIR to identify adulterated raw milk	PCA	5000 – 1000 cm^{-1}	FT-IR can be used to find out if milk has been adulterated with 0.05 and 0.075% sodium bicarbonate or citrate respectively.	Cassoli *et al.*, 2011
FTIR detection of melamine adulteration in milk	PLS	4000–650 cm^{-1}	Melamine could be detected at concentrations as low as 2.5 ppm using FTIR in conjunction with partial least-squares models.	Jawaid *et al.*, 2013
Detection of beef fat adulteration in butter fat	PLS	1500-1000 cm^{-1}	2.42% beef fat adulteration could be detected in butter fat	Nurrulhidayah *et al.*, 2013
Detection and quantification of soymilk in cow–buffalo milk using FTIR	PCA	1472–1241 cm^{-1}	0.92 for calibration and validation, respectively, can estimate the soya milk level in milk within the range of 1472–1241 cm-1.	Jaiswal *et al.*, 2015

Applications Significant	Chemometric technique used	Wavelength Used	Results	References
Detection of Fat and moisture contain in butter	MLR	3000–1000 cm^{-1}	FTIR can be applied for online process monitoring. The procedure required 20 seconds for sample analysis.	Upadhyay *et al.*, 2011
Detection of pig body fat in ghee	PCA, PLS	4000–500 cm^{-1}	Different absorption values were found for pure ghee, pig body fat, and pig body fat that had been added to pure ghee. This showed that ATR-FTIR can be used to find pig body fat in pure ghee.	Upadhyay *et al.*, 2018
Detection of goat body fat in ghee	PCA, PLS	4000–500 cm^{-1}	The different ways that pure ghee, goat body fat, and pure ghee with goat body fat absorbed light in certain spectral regions showed that FTIR and PLS can be used to determine adulterants in ghee.	Upadhyay *et al.*, 2016
Detection of corn starch, sodium bicarbonate, formaldehyde, saccharose, and sodium citrate in milk	PCA, PLS	5000-900 cm^{-1}	FTIR is a suitable replacement for identifying adulteration because it has been used in a number of industries to determine the composition of milk.	Coitinho *et al.*, 2017
Detection of Aflatoxin M1 in milk	PCA, PLS	4000–500 cm^{-1}	Variations in spectral areas were observed in the spectral window of 423–1123 and 3550–3499 cm1 when comparing pure milk samples to milk samples that had been spiked. A developed method was able to detect aflatoxin M1 in milk at concentrations as low as 0.02 g/l.	Jaiswal *et al.*, 2018
Detection of Formalin in cow milk	PCA, PLS	4000–400 cm^{-1}	FTIR method can detect 0.5% level of formalin in cow milk	Balan *et al.*, 2020
Detection of urea in milk	PCA, PLS	4000–700 cm^{-1}	FTIR approach able to detect 100 ppm of urea in milk.	Jha *et al.*, 2015

Advantages of Fourier Transform Infrared Spectroscopy

Speed

The majority of FT-IR measurements are made in a matter of seconds rather than several minutes because all of the frequencies are measured simultaneously.

Sensitivity

There are a number of different reasons why FT-IR results in a significant increase in sensitivity. The detectors that are used are significantly more sensitive, the optical throughput is significantly higher, which results in significantly lower noise levels, and the fast scans make it possible to perform multiple scans in order to reduce the random measurement noise to any level that is desired. It a very reliable technique for positive identification of virtually any sample.

Mechanical Simplicity

The only part of the interferometer that moves all the time is the moving mirror. So, there isn't much chance that the machine will break down.

Internally Calibrated

In order to achieve accurate measurement of wavelength, these instruments make use of a He-Ne laser as their internal standard. These instruments are self-calibrating, so the user will never have to worry about having to calibrate them.

This method is very reliable and can be used to positively identify any sample.

- The benefits of sensitivity make it possible to find even the smallest contaminants. Because of this, FT-IR is a very useful tool for quality control and quality assurance, whether it's comparing batches to quality standards or figuring out what a contaminant is.
- Also, the accuracy and sensitivity of FT-IR detectors, along with a wide range of software algorithms, have made it much easier to use infrared for quantitative analysis.
- Simple procedures for routine analysis can be adapted to include quantitative methods that are straightforward to develop and calibrate.
- There is only one moving part, so maintenance is easy.

Conclusion

FTIR spectroscopy is a versatile technique for identifying functional groups, studying macronutrients, and detecting several adulterants and impurities in foods. Coupled with chemometrics, it is a less difficult and more effective technology that has the potential to solve several industrial difficulties. However, it is a difficult task to select the appropriate statistical tool, as each method is designed to handle a distinct issue relative to FTIR-obtained spectra. This chapter has, however, attempted to detail and discuss the sequence of chemometric approaches that must be utilized, as well as the fundamental nature of each method and the problem it aims to solve. Consequently, if the optimal chemometric tool is applied to the spectra, this may resolve a number of issues confronting the food industry and researchers, such as the identification of their raw samples with regard to quality and safety, as FTIR coupled with chemometrics is a reasonably intelligent choice.

References

Araujo, M. C. U., Saldanha, T. C. B., Galvao, R. K. H., Yoneyama, T., Chame, H. C., & Visani, V., (2001). The successive projections algorithm for variable selection in spectroscopic multicomponent analysis. *Chemometrics and Intelligent Laboratory Systems, 57*(2), 65–73.

Balan, B., Dhaulaniya, A. S., Jamwal, R., Sodhi, K. K., Kelly, S., Cannavan, A., & Singh, D. K., (2020). Application of attenuated total reflectance-Fourier transform infrared (ATR-FTIR) spectroscopy coupled with chemometrics for detection and quantification of formalin in cow milk. *Vibrational Spectroscopy*, 107(103033), 1–7.

Barnes, R. J., Dhanoa, M. S., & Lister, S. J., (1993). Correction of the description of standard normal variate (SNV) and de-trend transformations in practical spectroscopy with applications in food and beverage analysis. *Journal of Near Infrared Spectroscopy*, 1, 185–186.

Blanco, M., Coello, J., Montoliu, I., & Romero, M. A., (2001). Orthogonal signal correction in near-infrared calibration. *Analytica Chimica Acta*, 434(1), 125–132.

Bureau, S., Ruiz, D., Reich, M., Gouble, B., Bertrand, D., Audergon, J. M., & Renard, C. M., (2009). Application of ATR-FTIR for a rapid and simultaneous determination of sugars and organic acids in apricot fruit. *Food Chemistry*, 115(3), 1133–1140.

Camacho, J., SMilde, A. K., Saccenti, E., & Westerhuis, J. A., (2019). All sparse PCA models are wrong, but some are useful. Part I: Computation of Scores, Residuals, and Explained Variance. (Accessed on 15 July 2022).

Cassoli, L. D., Sartori, B., Zampar, A., & Machado, P. F. (2011). An assessment of Fourier transform infrared spectroscopy to identify adulterated raw milk in Brazil. *International Journal of Dairy Technology*, 64(4), 480-485.

Coitinho, T. B., Cassoli, L. D., Cerqueira, P. H. R., Da Silva, H. K., Coitinho, J. B., & Machado, P. F., (2017). Adulteration identification in raw milk using Fourier transform infrared spectroscopy. *Journal of Food Science and Technology*, 54(8), 2394–2402.

Downey, G., Briandet, R., Wilson, R. H., & Kemsley, E. K., (1997). Near-and mid-infrared spectroscopies in food authentication: Coffee varietal identification. *Journal of Agricultural and Food Chemistry*, 45(11), 4357–4361.

Granato, D., Putnik, P., Kovačević, D. B., Santos, J. S., Calado, V., Rocha, R. S., Cruz, A. G. D., et al., (2018). Trends in chemometrics: Food authentication, microbiology, and effects of processing. *Comprehensive Reviews in Food Science and Food Safety*, 17(3), 663–677.

Hacisalihoglu, G., Larbi, B., & Mark, S. A., (2010). Near-infrared reflectance spectroscopy predicts protein, starch, and seed weight in intact seeds of common bean (*Phaseolus Vulgaris* L.). *Journal of Agricultural and Food Chemistry, 58*(2), 702–706.

Haghiri, M., (2016). Consumer choice between food safety and food quality: The case of farm-raised Atlantic salmon. *Foods*, 5(2), 22–29.

Jaiswal, P., Jha, S. N., Borah, A., Gautam, A., Grewal, M. K., & Jindal, G., (2015). Detection and quantification of soymilk in cow-buffalo milk using attenuated total reflectance Fourier transform infrared spectroscopy (ATR-FTIR). *Food Chemistry*, 168, 41–47.

Jaiswal, P., Jha, S. N., Kaur, J., Borah, A., & Ramya, H. G., (2018). Detection of aflatoxin M1 in milk using spectroscopy and multivariate analyses. *Food Chemistry*, 238, 209–214.

Jawaid, S., Talpur, F. N., Sherazi, S. T. H., Nizamani, S. M., & Khaskheli, A. A. (2013). Rapid detection of melamine adulteration in dairy milk by SB-ATR–Fourier transform infrared spectroscopy. *Food chemistry*, 141(3), 3066-3071.

Jha, S. N., Jaiswal, P., Borah, A., Gautam, A. K., & Srivastava, N., (2015). Detection and quantification of urea in milk using attenuated total Reflectance-Fourier transform infrared spectroscopy. *Food and Bioprocess Technology, 8*(4), 926–933.

Jolliffe, I. T., & Cadima, J., (2016). Principal component analysis: A review and recent developments. Philosophical Transactions of the Royal Society A: *Mathematical, Physical and Engineering Sciences*, 374(2065), 20150202.

Justice, A. C., Covinsky, K. E., & Berlin, J. A., (1999). Assessing the generalizability of prognostic information. *Annals Internal Medicine*, 130(6), 515–524.

Keshavarzi, Z., Banadkoki, S. B., Faizi, M., Zolghadri, Y., & Shirazi, F. H., (2020). Comparison of transmission FTIR and ATR Spectra for discrimination between beef and chicken meat and quantification of chicken in beef meat mixture using ATR-FTIR combined with chemometrics. *Journal of Food Science and Technology*, 57(4), 1430–1438.

Kohonen, T., (1995). *Self-Organizing Maps* (1st edn., p. 362). Berlin, Germany: Springer.

Lee, L. C., Liong, C. Y., & Jemain, A. A., (2017). A contemporary review on data preprocessing (DP) practice strategy in ATR-FTIR spectrum. *Chemometrics and Intelligent Laboratory Systems*, 163, 64–75.

Leite, A. I. N., Pereira, C. G., Andrade, J., Vicentini, N. M., Bell, M. J. V., & Anjos, V., (2019). FTIR-ATR spectroscopy as a tool for the rapid detection of adulterations in butter cheeses. *LWT-Food Science and Technology*, 109, 63–69.

Liu, L., Wang, Y., Gao, C., Huan, H., Zhao, B., & Yan, L., (2015). Photoacoustic spectroscopy as a non-destructive tool for quantification of pesticide residue in apple cuticle. *International Journal of Thermophysics*, 36(5–6), 868–872.

Lv, G., Du, C., Ma, F., Shen, Y., & Zhou, J., (2018). Rapid and non-destructive detection of pesticide residues by depth-profiling Fourier transform infrared photoacoustic spectroscopy. *ACS Omega*, 3(3), 3548–3553.

Nicolaou, N., & Goodacre, R. (2008). Rapid and quantitative detection of the microbial spoilage in milk using Fourier transform infrared spectroscopy and chemometrics. *Analyst,* 133(10), 1424-1431.

Nicolaou, N., Xu, Y., & Goodacre, R. (2010). Fourier transform infrared spectroscopy and multivariate analysis for the detection and quantification of different milk species. *Journal of dairy scienc*e, 93(12), 5651-5660.

Nurrulhidayah, A. F., Che Man, Y. B., Rohman, A., Amin, I., Shuhaimi, M., &Khatib, A. (2013). Authentication analysis of butter from beef fat using Fourier Transform Infrared (FTIR) spectroscopy coupled with chemometrics. *International Food Research Journal*, 20 (3), 1383-1388.

Paradkar, M. M., &Irudayaraj, J. (2002). Determination of cholesterol in dairy products using infrared techniques: 1. FTIR spectroscopy. *International Journal of Dairy Technology*, 55(3), 127-132.

Ranvir, S., Gandhi, K., & Sharma, N. (2018). Fourier Transform Infrared Spectroscopy–Concept and its Application in Quality Assessment of Dairy Foods. *Centre of Advanced Faculty Training in Dairy Processing.*

Sahu, D. K., Rai, J., Rai, M. K., Nirmal, M., Wani, K., Banjare, M. K., & Mundeja, P., (2020). Detection of flonicamid insecticide in vegetable samples by UV-visible spectrophotometer and FTIR. *Results in Chemistry*, 100059.

Settle, F. A., (1997). *Handbook of Instrumental Techniques for Analytical Chemistry* (pp. 56, 57). Prentice-Hall, Upper Saddle River; New Jersey; USA.

Silverstein, R. M., Webster, F. X., Kiemle, D. J., & Bryce, D. L., (2014). Spectrometric Identification of Organic Compounds (8th edn., pp. 71–76). New Jersey, USA: Wiley.

Stuart, B. H., (2000). Infrared spectroscopy. In: Meyers, R. A., (ed.), *Encyclopedia of Analytical Chemistry* (pp. 529–559). Chichester, UK: John Wiley & Sons, Inc.

Stuart, B. H., (2004). Infrared Spectroscopy: Fundamentals and Applications (pp. 15–37). London-UK: John Wiley and Sons.

Sun, D. W., (2009). Infrared Spectroscopy for Food Quality Analysis and Control (pp. 8–11). Burlington, USA: Academic Press.

Upadhyay, N., Goyal, A., & Rathod, G., (2011). Microwave spectroscopy and its applications in online processing. *Indian Food Industry*, 30(5/6), 63–73.

Upadhyay, N., Jaiswal, P., & Jha, S. N., (2016). Detection of goat body fat adulteration in pure ghee using ATR-FTIR spectroscopy coupled with chemometric strategy. *Journal of Food Science and Technology*, 53(10), 3752–3760.

Upadhyay, N., Jaiswal, P., & Jha, S. N., (2018). Application of attenuated total reflectance Fourier transform infrared spectroscopy (ATR–FTIR) in MIR range coupled with chemometrics for detection of pig body fat in pure ghee (heat clarified milk fat). *Journal of Molecular Structure*, 1153, 275–281.

Yang, H., & Irudayaraj, J., (2002). Rapid determination of vitamin C by NIR, MIR, and FT-Raman techniques. *Journal of Pharmacy and Pharmacology*, 54(9), 1247–1255.

Ye, J., (2007). Least Squares Linear Discriminant Analysis, 7. http://staff.ustc.edu. cn/~zwp/teach/MVA/icml2007_Ye07.pdf (Accessed on 15 July 2022).

8

Applications of Enzyme Based Flavour Components in Dairy Products

Partha Pratim Debnath[1], Anindita Debnath[2], Kuntal Roy[3] Payal Karmakar[4], Ronit Mandal[5] and Jimi Roy Sarkar[6]

[1]*Faculty of Dairy Technology, West Bengal University of Animal and Fishery Sciences (WBUAFS), Mohanpur, Nadia, West Bengal, India*
[2]*Faculty of Dairy Technology, WBUAFS, Mohanpur, Nadia, West Bengal India*
[3]*Faculty of Dairy Technology, WBUAFS, Mohanpur, Nadia, West Bengal India*
[4]*Division of Diary Chemistry, National Dairy Research Institute, Karnal Haryana, India*
[5]*Faculty of Land and Food systems, University of British Columbia, Vancouver-V6T1Z4, British Columbia, Canada*
[6]*Food Safety Officer, Dakshin Dinajpur, West Bengal, India*

Abstract

Flavour is a prominent attribute for consumer acceptability of any dairy product. Various additives have been used to improve or enhance the flavour. But recently, due to higher consumer preference of natural flavours as compared to synthetic flavours, there is a considerable increase in the utilization of enzymes for flavour enhancement in various dairy products. Lipase, protease and esterase enzyme has been used extensively for increasing the flavour intensity of various dairy products. In addition to this, enzymes are also being used to impart dairy flavour (e.g. cheese flavour) in various other food products. This chapter will mainly deal with various sources of enzymes used and their specificity and mechanism of action. Also, this chapter will focus upon the pathways by which enzyme synthesizes the various flavouring compounds in dairy products. The applications of the enzyme modified flavourings in different dairy products will also be discussed in details here.

Introduction

Enzymes (biological catalyst) can be defined as a substance which initiates or fastens the reaction rate, without being consumed during the reaction. Enzymes function as a catalyst in various biological processes taking place in all life forms. Although enzyme synthesis takes place inside living cells, they can even function as a catalyst in the *in vitro* processes, which makes it suitable for many industrial applications. For product formation in any chemical reaction, reactants or substrates has to overcome the transition state. This energy required to achieve the transition state is known as activation energy. Enzymes or catalyst accelerate the reaction rate by reducing this activation energy (Blanco and Blanco, 2017). The enzyme activity is represented in enzyme units or international units (IU) or katals (Kat). The quantity of enzyme required for catalyzing the conversion of 1μM of substrate/ minute under optimum conditions (pH, temperature etc.) is being described as 1 IU. The enzyme activity is affected by temperature, pH, concentration of substrate, amount of enzyme and also by enzyme activators or inhibitors. As compared to many inorganic catalysts, enzymes are more efficient and are also highly specific or selective. In addition, enzymes can be recycled and reused without any loss of activity by immobilization technique. Dr. James B. Summer is being credited for the first isolation of the enzyme urease, in crystalline form from jack bean (Kuddus, 2019). Most of the enzymes are protein in nature. The enzymes are being subdivided into six broad classes i.e. oxidoreductases, transferases, hydrolases, lyases, isomerases and ligases.

Enzymes (specifically microbial source) have diversified applications in sectors like agriculture, pharmaceutical, food, energy and chemicals. The usage of enzymes in food industry dates back to 6000 BCE, when Sumerians and Babylonians used microorganisms from barley yeast for industrial production of alcoholic beverages (Abada, 2019). Rennet has been used as a coagulating enzyme in dairy sector since 6000 BCE. In dairy industry, enzymes of microbial source are remarkably used for coagulation, accelerated cheese ripening, protein cross linking and for flavour enhancement. Depending upon the taste and flavour perception, consumer's food preferences vary. Flavour is considered a blend of three senses i.e. taste, smell and chemosensory irritation (Beauchamp and Mennella, 2009). The global flavour market in 2007 stood at USD 8.45 billion, of which food flavours accounted 25% share with about 5% annual growth rate (Guentert, 2007; Christen and Lopez Munguia, 1991).The flavour enhancement of dairy products increases the consumer satisfaction and its acceptability. Synthetic dairy flavours are widely available, but natural dairy flavours are gaining huge importance due to health concerns. Natural flavouring materials are those which are derived by suitable physical, enzymatic and microbiological methods, from plant or animal sources and the flavouring materials may be in raw form or processed form for human consumption (Gandhi, 1997). In dairy products, break down components of milk protein and fat, are considered as the main sources of flavour generation. This degradation of milk protein and fat for flavour generation can be achieved by incorporating enzymes. Mostly lipase, protease and esterase are used in dairy industry for flavour enhancement, which will be discussed in details in this chapter.

Sources of Enzymes

Though enzymes are present in all living organisms, but commercial enzymes are derived from three basic sources, i.e. animals, micro-organisms and plants. However, microbial enzymes is the most preferred source for industrial usage because of i) lower production cost, ii) widely available raw materials having steady composition for microbial growth, iii) environment friendly and non-toxic in nature, iv) cost effective in final usage. By application of recombinant DNA technology, microbes can be altered to produce enzyme which fulfils the desirable attributes in finished product. In 2014, the global market of microbial enzymes stood at USD 4.2 billion and a 7% market growth is expected by 2020 (Abada, 2019).

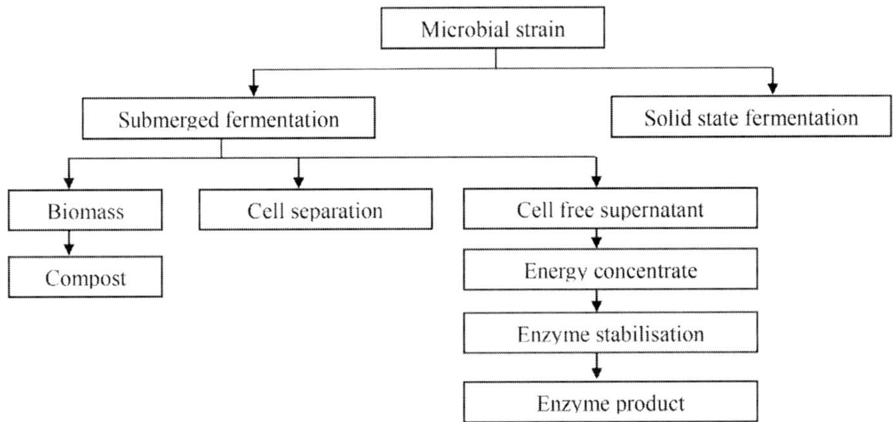

Fig. 8.1: Manufacturing of microbial enzymes
(*Source*: Abada, 2019)

In dairy sector, microbial enzymes lead to improvement and enhancement of organoleptic properties (colour, flavour, aroma and texture), along with an increase in yield of dairy products. Microbial enzymes have been used in yoghurt, cheese, butter, butter oil, ghee, anhydrous milk fat and paneer for quality enhancement (Table 8.1).

Table 8.1: Usage of enzymes in dairy sector

Enzyme	Dairy product	Function	Micro-organisms
Aminopeptidase	Cheese	Accelerated ripening	*Lactobacillus sp.*
Rennet	Cheese	Milk coagulation	*Aspergillus sp., Rhizomucor sp.*
Catalase	Cheese	Processing	*Aspergillus niger*
Lipase	Cheese	Accelerated ripening and flavour development	*Aspergillus niger*
Neutral proteinase	Cheese	Accelerated ripening and flavour enhancement	*Bacillus sp., Aspergillus oryzae*
Transglutaminase	Cheese and paneer	Protein cross linking	*Streptomyces sp.*
Lipase	Enzyme Modified Ghee Flavour	Flavour enhancement	*Rhizopus oryzae*
Protease	Enzyme Modified Ghee Flavour	Flavour enhancement	*Aspergillus sp.*
Esterase	Cheese	Flavour enhancement	*Mucor miehei*

Lipases in Flavour Development in Dairy Industry

The indigenous lipase enzyme in milk hydrolyses the milk fat and produces fatty acids. Extensive hydrolysis of milk fat imparts rancid flavour to dairy products. Thermal treatment restricts the rancid flavour development by inactivating the native lipase enzyme. However, controlled lipolysis of milk fat is desirable in few products and thus lipase enzyme (externally added) is extensively used for flavour enhancement in products like cheese, ghee, anhydrous milk fat etc. Lipase enzyme belongs to hydrolases group and is responsible for cleaving the triacylglycerol of milk fat to produce diacylglycerol and free fatty acids (FFA), in aqueous environment (Figure 8.2). However, non-aqueous environment during lipolysis, paves the way for glycerides formation from glycerol and fatty acids by esterification reaction.

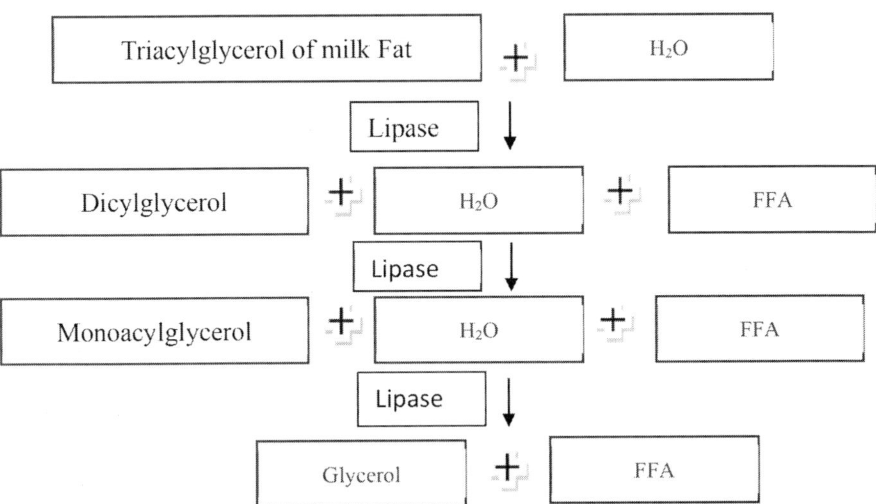

Fig. 8.2: Hydrolysis of milk fat by lipase enzyme
(*Source*: Kumar and Ray, 2014)

Lipases derived from different sources have varied enzymatic specificity. Few lipases are more specific to fatty acids having short chain length (acetic acid, butyric acid, caproic and capric acid), but some lipases have higher affinity for unsaturated fatty acids (oleic acid, linoleic and linolenic acid) (Jooyandeh *et al*., 2009). Although, certain lipases are not specific in nature. Lipases also exhibit stereo-specificity i.e. they are capable to distinguish between the sn-1 and sn-3 position of triacylglycerols (Kontkanen *et al.*, 2014). Lipases preferably attack the fatty acids at sn-1 and sn-3 position and not the sn-2 position. Therefore, the end products of a lipolytic reaction will depend upon the type of lipase enzyme used and its specificity. Short chain fatty acids (SCFA) (at sn-3 position) are the most important flavour contributors followed by medium chain and long chain fatty acid (LCFA) (Figure 8.3). SCFA imparts desired buttery flavours whereas LCFA produces undesirable soapy or bitter flavour. Thus, lipase enzyme having sn-1, 3 specificity (mostly hydrolyzing SCFA) should be used for flavour enhancement of dairy products.

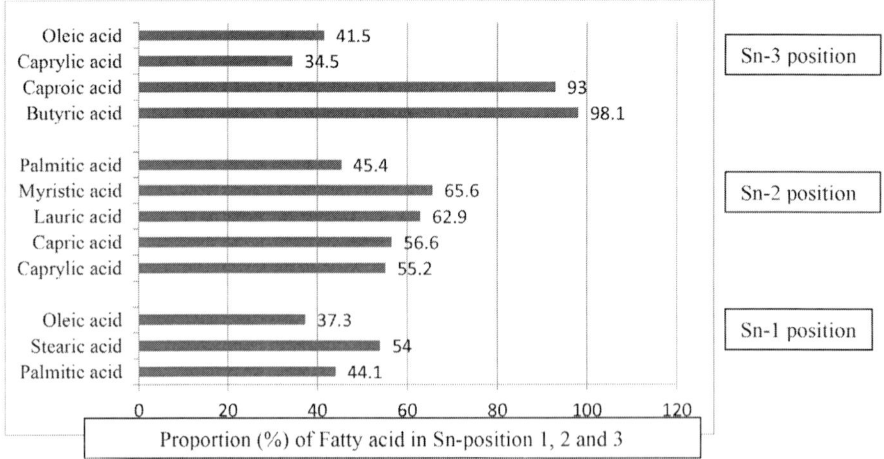

Fig. 8.3: Sn-position of major fatty acids present in milk fat
(*Source*: Jensen, 2002)

Lipase activity is dependent upon the quantity of oil found at the interface as lipase works at oil-water interface (Jooyandeh *et al.*, 2009; Kontkanen *et al.*, 2014). Agitation and emulsifier addition increases the interfacial area and as a result increases the lipase activity. The various flavouring compounds originating from the hydrolysis of milk fat by lipase enzyme are methyl ketones, free fatty acids (FFA), lactones, aldehydes, acids and alcohols (Figure 8.4).

Esterases in Flavour Development in Dairy Industry

Esterase belongs to the class of hydrolases and is responsible for catalyzing the hydrolysis of esters in milk fat. Three native esterase enzyme are present in milk, named as A, B and C. An esterase splits aromatic esters (phenyl acetate), B- esterase cleaves aliphatic and aromatic esters and C–esters hydrolyses the choline esters (Dwivedi *et al.*, 2009). The B-esterase exhibits similar properties to lipase as it can hydrolyse the glyecrol. Also, the mechanism of hydrolysis of esterases is very similar to lipases. Never the less, there are certain differences between lipase and esterase. The differentiation is based upon the physico chemical nature of substrates on which the enzymes act and the fatty acids chain length in the substrates. The esterases can perform the hydrolysis reaction only in aqueous solutions and it can split only fatty acids having short chain length. Water soluble substrates are more preferred by esterases (Jaeger and Reetz, 1998). However, lipases work at oil water interface and it can hydrolyse both long and short chain fatty acids. Water insoluble substrates are more preferred by lipases. The native milk esterases are soluble at pH 4.6, therefore during cheese preparation very less proportion of esterases are present in cheese curd as most of it are lost in whey (Kitchen, 1971). Thus, esterase enzyme is externally incorporated in cheese such that optimum flavour development takes place during ripening. Esters provide a fruity flavour note in dairy products. The undesirable off flavours which are imparted by higher concentration of short chain FFA, can be masked by esters. However, excessive amount of ethyl esters can cause fruity flavour defect in milk products.

Proteases in Flavour Development in Dairy Industry

Proteinase (peptidase) is the term used for the enzymes which hydrolyses the proteins in milk to form large peptides. The peptides and amino acids liberated during the proteolysis reaction, act as flavour precursors. The native protease enzyme in milk is present in very small quantity. The indigenous protease enzyme exhibits tryptic and chymotryptic substrate specificity, but is inhibited by di-isopropyl fluoro phosphate (Kaminogawa *et al.,* 1969). Protease has varied enzymatic specificity. Few protease enzymes are more specific to certain amino acids like aspartic acid, glutamic acid, cysteine, serine and threonine. But, some proteases require metal ions for enzymatic activity (Nunez, 2016). Amino-proteases, tri-proteases, endo-proteases, extra cellular proteases and serine proteases fall in the group of proteolytic proteases (Quereshi *et al*., 2015). Amino-proteases perform a crucial part in flavour enhancement of dairy products as they hydrolyse large oligopeptides into amino acids having single residues. Proteases are used to reduce bitterness as it degrades the hydrophobic amino acids in various dairy products.

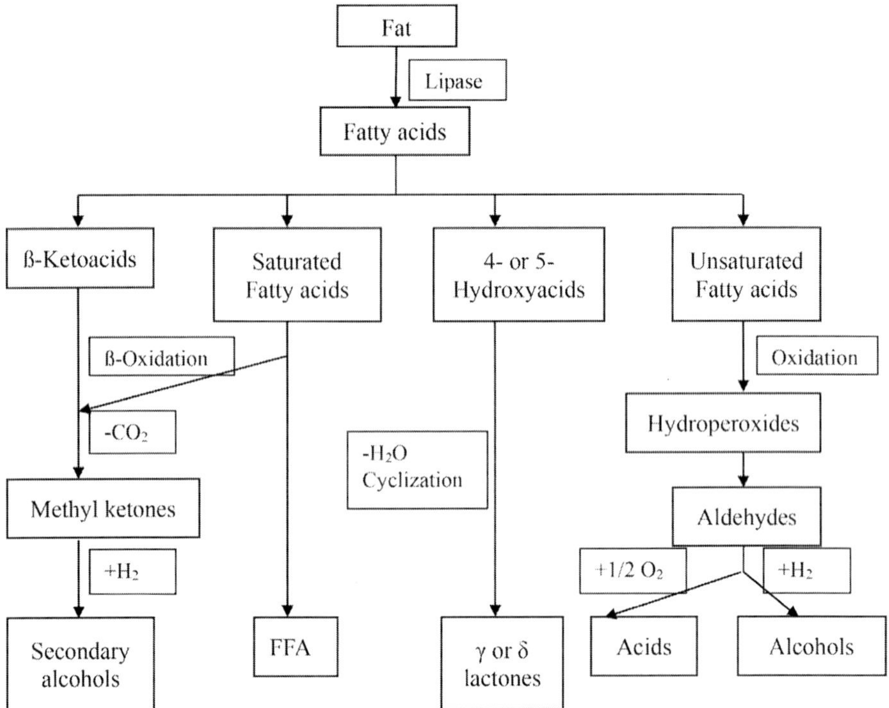

Fig. 8.4: Synthesis of flavouring compounds from milk fat by lipase enzyme (*Source*: Dumont and Adda, 1978)

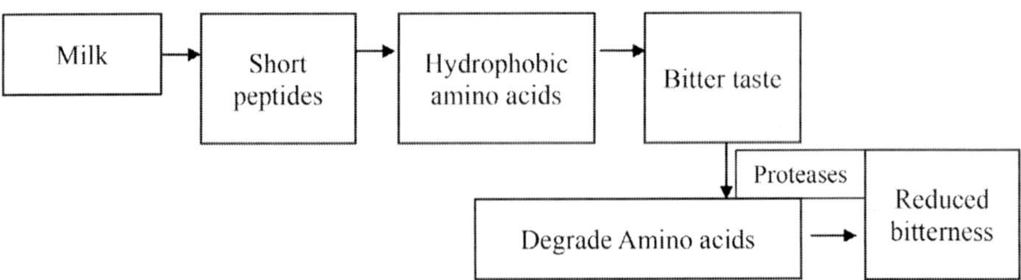

Fig. 8.5: Reduction of bitter taste by proteases in dairy products (Abada, 2019)

The ß-casein fraction is the most sensitive to proteolysis, which is followed by αs- and k casein. Proteolysis does not take place in raw milk under normal environment (in absence of proteolytic bacteria), even though the native protease enzyme is bonded with k-casein in milk. Therefore, protease enzyme is externally added in dairy products to enhance its flavour by controlled proteolysis. The various flavouring compounds obtained from milk protein by proteases involve acetophenone, amines, α-keto acids, aldehydes, alcohols, acids, phenol, cresol, indole and methional (Figure 8.6).

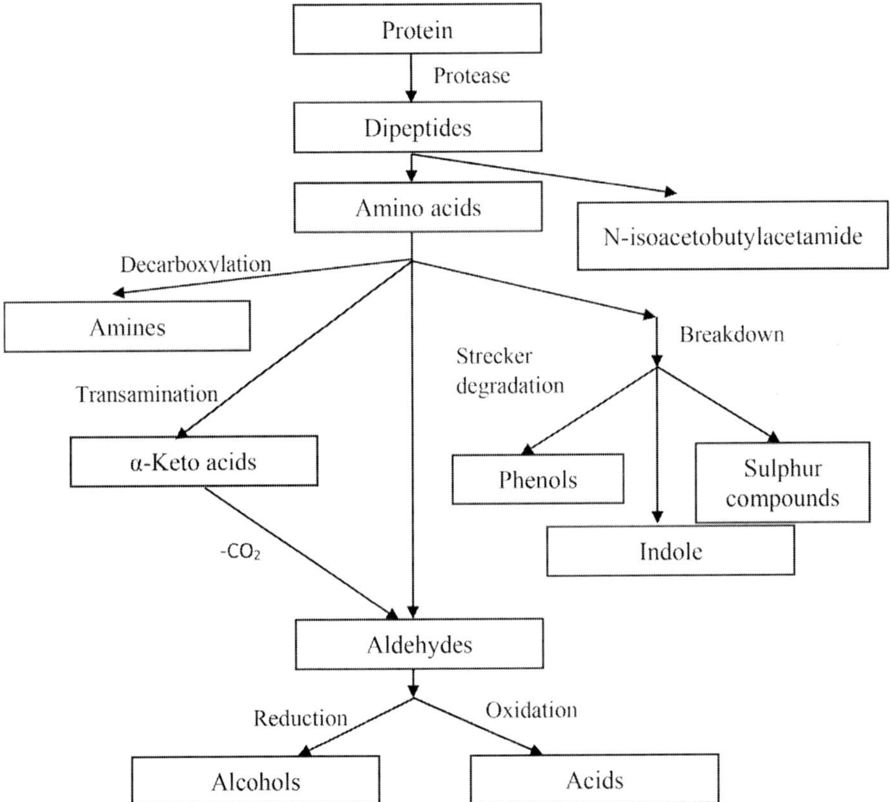

Fig. 8.6: Synthesis of flavour compounds by protein degradation with protease enzyme (Dumont and Adda, 1978)

Proteinase Plasmin (PL) also plays a pivotal role in flavour development of milk products. The native plasmin in milk is found in zymogen form, inactive plasminogen (PG). PG can be transformed into PL by plasminogen activators (tissue type and urokinase type) (Figure 8.7). The PL system components interact with each other and other parts, for example, whey and casein, and either promote or inhibit proteolysis. Among all the casein fractions in milk, k-casein is only not subjected to plasmin activity. Plasmin enzyme has been added in Emmental, Gouda and Cheddar cheese to enhance it flavour during ripening (Farkye and Fox, 1991).

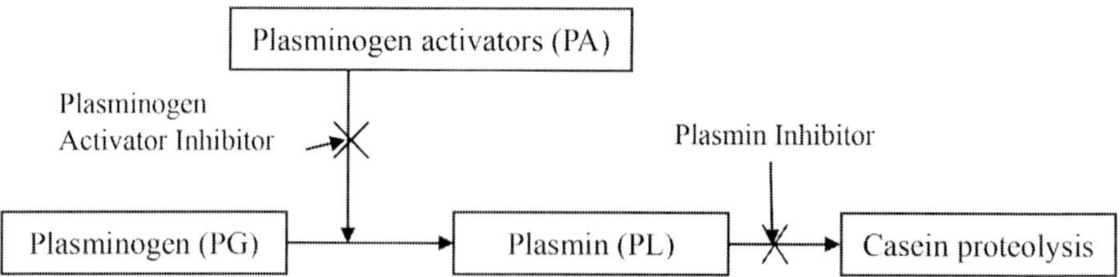

Fig. 8.7: Plasmin enzyme system in milk and proteolysis of casein (Ismail and Nielsen, 2010)

Incorporation of Enzymes in Milk Products

Exogenous enzymes can be added i) with milk before cheese production and with cream or butter during enzyme modified ghee manufacture, ii) along with starter culture/ coagulant during cheese manufacture, iii) during dry salting of cheese, iv) with curd slurries, v) directly within cheese block or ghee, vi) enzyme encapsulation, vii) enzyme immobilization.

Phospholipase and proteinase *(Pseudomonas fluorescens)* has been added in milk before cheese manufacture for flavour enhancement in Cheddar cheese. Urokinase has been supplemented in milk to increase the activity of plasmin before Havarti and Cheddar cheese production for accelerated proteolysis and flavour development (Wilkinson and Kilcawley, 2005). Protease and lipase enzyme has also been incorporated in cream and butter directly during enzyme modified ghee (EMG) manufacture for intensifying the ghee flavour (Debnath and Ghosh, 2018). In EMG, enzymes after mixing with small amount of water have also been directly added to ghee for flavour enhancement.

Proteinase enzyme is also added in milk along with rennet or starter culture in cheese. But this method of enzyme addition prematurely splits the casein and therefore interferes with rennet coagulation and decreases cheese yield. In addition, ninety percent of the enzyme gets lost in whey during separation of whey from cheese curd (Wilkinson and Kilcawley, 2005). In order to reduce the enzyme losses in whey, enzymes are blended during the dry salting of cheese. However, the principal limitation in this method is the uniform distribution of small quantity of enzyme into large amount of curd. The enzymatic action in this method is dependent on the extent of diffusion, which is affected by the molecule size, charge, structure and its conformation and the enzyme specificity. Incorporation of enzymes into brine salted cheeses may be more difficult and is dependent upon the solubility of enzymes (Wilkinson and Kilcawley, 2005).

Enzymes are also mixed during cheese production by utilising curd slurries. Curd slurries are prepared by blending grated cheese curd and water, followed by emulsification to 40-60% moisture and finally incubating it for one to seven days. Enzymes are usually incorporated before the incubation of curd slurries. Curd slurries can be added in cheese both in wet or dried form and in pasteurized or unpasteurized form. Curd slurries can be added at varying stages of cheese manufacture i) directly in milk along with starter, ii) directly into cheese curd before Cheddaring, iii) directly during dry salting before milling (best method). Accelerated ripening and flavour development has been observed in Cheddar cheese by adding spray dried curd slurry or enzyme modified cheese (EMC) directly into cheese curd during dry salting , before milling (Wilkinson and Kilcawley, 2005). Enzymes in aqueous form have been directly injected into Mozzarella cheese block by using high pressure injector. Higher fluid pressure and velocity, higher penetration by needle and higher temperature (above 43°C) of cheese block will improve the retention of enzyme in cheese.

Enzyme encapsulation method is used to protect the enzymes form exterior environment and for controlled release of enzymes. Enzymes has been encapsulated in milk fat fractions, cold melting hydrogel beads, food gums (agar, carrageenan, alginate etc.) and liposomes. Encapsulation of enzymes by the liposomes is the most effective method as they are manufactured from components naturally found in cheese and they prevent pre-mature hydrolysis of casein during cheese preparation. The efficiency obtained by encapsulating enzyme with liposome is ninety six percent, along with sixty four percent enzyme entrapments in curd (Wilkinson and Kilcawley, 2005). The enzyme entrapment in curd is affected by type of liposome and phospholipid, method of cheese manufacturing and the type of enzyme to be encapsulated. The enzyme release from liposomes is controlled by temperature, pH, ionic concentration and phospholipase. Immobilization of lipase enzyme with *Yarrowia lipolytica* cell debris has been carried out to manufacture lipolysed milk fat (LMF). This LMF can be used to impart or enhance flavour in various dairy products. In this method, the enzyme has been reused four times. The lipolytic activity after second time usage of enzyme has been observed seventy percent and it reduces to forty percent after the fourth time usage (Fraga *et al.*, 2018).

Flavour Enhancement of Cheese by Enzymes

According to Food Safety Standards authority of India (FSSAI), 2017 cheese is derived from complete or partial coagulation of protein, which is obtained from milk, skimmed milk, partly skimmed milk, cream, whey cream or buttermilk or mixture of these materials, with the help of suitable enzymes of non-animal origin or other suitable coagulating agents, with or without use of harmless lactic acid bacteria and by partially draining the whey resulting from the coagulation. Cheese may be either ripened or un-ripened. Flavour generation in cheese occurs mainly during ripening by three pathways i.e. proteolysis, lipolysis and glycolysis. Incorporation of lipase, esterase and protease enzyme in cheese catalyses the proteolysis and lipolysis process, leading to flavour enhancement and accelerated ripening. The flavouring compounds identified in cheese are methylbutanal, methanethiol, dimethylsulphide, methional, benzaldehyde, methylpropanol, butyric acid, acetic acid, butanone, hexanal, pentanal, γ-decalactone, ethyl butyrate and ethyl hexanonate (Hassan *et al.*, 2012). Commerical lipase, protease (including plasmin) and esterase enzyme has been used for flavour development of Cheddar cheese (Nunez, 2016), Manchego type cheese (Garcia *et al.*, 1994), Italian cheeses (Romano and provolone) and Mozzarella cheese, Feta cheese and Blue cheese (Jooyandeh *et al.*, 2009).

Lipase and protease has been extensively used in the preparation of enzyme modified cheese (EMC) flavourings (Wilkinson and Kilcawley, 2003). EMC is prepared by incubating cheese curd with lipase and protease enzyme at high temperature (30-45°C), such that an intensified cheese flavour is produced, which can be successively used in various food products like processed cheese, analogue cheese, cheese spreads and dips, bakery products and in foods having low fat. EMC are advantageous over other synthetic or natural cheese flavours because of higher flavour intensity (ten times higher FFA than green cheese), easy availability of wide varieties of flavour (Swiss, Gouda, Mozzarella and Cheddar cheese flavour), lower production costs, higher shelf life and also, very less quantity (0.1% w/w) of EMC is required to impart cheese flavour. EMC flavour (if dried) can be dry blended to impart cheesy flavour in biscuits and snacks.

Flavour Enhancement of Ghee by Enzymes

Ghee is defined as the pure clarified milk fat. Ghee has a pleasant, slightly cooked and caramalised flavour. The flavour of ghee is mainly influenced by clarification temperature of ghee, bacterial hydrolysis (ripening) and enzymatic hydrolysis of cream or butter. The major flavouring compounds in ghee are free fatty acid (FFA), carbonyls, lactones, esters, ketones, aldehydes, alcohols and diols. Lipase and protease enzyme has been used for the production of enzyme modified ghee (EMG) flavour (Debnath and Ghosh, 2018). EMG flavour is prepared by using lipase and protease enzyme (3:1) (@ 0.05%) in combination on ghee/ butter/ cream (substrates) at elevated temperature

(45°C) for 180 minutes to produce intensified ghee flavour (4 times intense flavour as compared to normal ghee). The enzymes are also inactivated by heat treatment to prevent extensive lipolysis and proteolysis. Ghee residue is also separated by filtration. Inactivation of enzymes added at cream and butter stage occurs during clarification of ghee. However, if the enzyme is added in ghee (as a substrate), it requires further heat treatment (80°C/10 minutes) after clarification for enzyme inactivation. EMG flavour, produced from enzyme addition in cream yields the best ghee flavour as sufficient water is available for enzymatic action, leading to better diffusion of enzymes and also, re-heating of ghee is not required (no loss of volatile flavours) for enzyme inactivation. The flavouring compounds identified in EMG are 5-(hydroxymethyl)-2-furancarboxyldehyde, butanal, benzeneacetaldehyde, undecanone, tri-decanone, nonanone, decanoic acid methyl ester, formic acid-1-methylethyl ester, acetic acid, butanoic acid, heptanoic acid, maltol, octanol etc (Debnath and Ghosh, 2018).

EMG flavour can be used in less quantity (as compared to normal ghee) in variety of food products like gulabjamun, jalebi etc. to impart the ghee flavour. EMG flavour can also be used as high aroma ghee as it satisfies all the FSSAI (Food Safety Standards authority of India) standards of ghee. Not only that ghee produced by this enzymatic treatment has a higher shelf life and higher yield as compared to normal ghee. The higher shelf life is mainly attributed to the formation of higher maillard reaction products (MRPs) which has oxygen radical absorbing capacity.

Flavour Enhancement of Anhydrous Milk Fat (AMF) by Enzymes

According to FSSAI (2017) anhydrous milk fat (AMF) is a fat rich product which is obtained solely from milk or milk products or both, by almost eliminating the water and milk solids not fat. Immobilized lipase enzyme (Lipozyme-435) derived from *Rhizomucor miehei*, has been used to hydrolyze AMF for flavour enhancement (Omar *et al.*, 2015). AMF has been hydrolyzed by using lipase enzyme along with phosphate buffer at 55°C for 12 hr. After hydrolysis, filter paper is used to separate the lipase enzyme from hydrolyzed AMF. The hydrolyzed AMF is then immediately subjected to centrifugation (2147g/10 minute) followed by top layer separation. It is then finally stored at -20°C. The flavouring compounds produced from AMF hydrolysis are butanoic acid, hexanoic acid, octanoic acid, heptanone, nonanone, benzaldehyde, phenol, acetaldehyde, dodecanoic acid, hexanoic acid, tetradecanoic acid etc. The hydrolyzed AMF is also used to enhance flavour in various dairy products like butter oil.

Other Applications of Enzymes in Flavour Enhancement

Apart from the above discussed products, lipolytic enzymes have also been used for production of enzyme modified milk powder, lipolysed milk, lipolysed milk fat "buttery" flavour, lipolysed milk fat "cultured cream" flavours, lipolysed milk fat "blue cheese" flavours, lipolysed milk fat "cheese-like" flavours and yoghurt (Seitz, 1990). But, as these are patented researches therefore very few details are available. In cultured dairy products, micro-organisms are used which degrades carbohydrates, fats and proteins for their survival. Flavour compounds like diacetyl, acetaldehyde etc. get generated as byproducts of the above metabolic processes, which is being catalyzed by the enzymes present in the micro-organism. Enzyme such as sulphydryl oxidase has been used to eliminate cooked flavour in sterilized or UHT (ultra high temperature processing) milk, by oxidizing the sulphydryl or thiol groups to disulfides.

Off Flavours Produced by Native Milk Enzymes

Milk peroxidase enzyme, also referred as lactoperoxidase, produces off flavours by oxidation of milk fat (Dwivedi *et al.*, 2009). Lactoperoxidase (LPO) is more heat stable as compared to other enzymes and it forms 1% of total whey protein. Hydrogen peroxide is mostly used as a hydrogen acceptor for peroxidases. Phenols and amines are generally the hydrogen donors. The oxidation reaction leads to the production of enzyme hydrogen donor complexes.

$LPO + H_2O_2 = \text{Complex A}$

$\text{Complex A} + RH_2 = \text{Complex B} + RH$

$\text{Complex B} + RH = LPO + R$

where, RH_2 is hydrogen donor and R is oxidized acceptor

Xanthine oxidase senzyme (also known as dehydrogenase) is also responsible for oxidized milk flavour (Dwivedi *et al.*, 2009). It leads to oxidation of purines, pyrimidines and aldehydes. Xanthine oxidase enzyme is a fairly heat stable and its enzymatic activity in milk increases with repeated heat treatments, homogenization and with the action of protease and lipase enzyme. Though lipase enzyme has been used in flavour enhancement of various dairy products, but if the native lipase enzyme undergoes extensive lipolysis it may lead to rancid flavour.

Conclusion

Enzymes obtained from microbial source are mostly used for flavour enhancement of dairy products. Lipase, protease and esterase enzymes are mainly utilized for increasing the flavour intensity in cheese (by hydrolyzing protein and fat) and also for reducing the ripening time. Lipase enzyme having specificity over short chain fatty acids (SCFA) should be chosen for flavour enhancement as SCFA are the most important flavour contributor. EMC flavour, EMG flavour and lipase hydrolyzed AMF can be used to impart cheese, ghee and milk fat flavour respectively in various food products. However, extensive lipolysis and proteolysis should be avoided to prevent the formation of off flavours. More researches have to be carried out to evaluate the economical feasibility of enzyme modified flavours for commercial operations, while keeping in mind the enzyme stability and production capacity. Thus, enzymatic mode of natural flavour formation or enhancement is an attractive and beneficial approach and it can be expected in future that, there will be more commercial applications of natural enzymatic flavours.

References

Abada, E. A. (2019). Application of microbial enzymes in the dairy industry. In *Enzymes in Food Biotechnology* (pp. 61-72). Academic Press.

Beauchamp, G. K., & Mennella, J. A. (2009). Early flavor learning and its impact on later feeding behavior. *Journal of Pediatric Gastroenterology and Nutrition*, *48*, S25-S30.

Blanco, A., & Blanco, G. (2017). Chapter 8—Enzymes. *Medical Biochemistry; Blanco, A., Blanco, G., Eds*, 153-175.

Christen, P., & López□Munguía, A. (1994). Enzymes and food flavor□A review. *Food Biotechnology*, 8(2-3), 167-190.

Debnath, P. P., & Ghosh, B. C. (2018). Enzyme Modified Ghee Flavour: Application and Shelf Life Studies. *Int. J. Pure App. Biosci*, 6(5), 822-826.

Dumont, J. P., & Adda, J. (1978, April). Flavour formation in dairy products. In *2. Weurmann Flavour Research Symposium*. Applied Science Publishers.

Dwivedi, B. K., Shahani, K. M., & Arnold, R. G. (2009). The role of enzymes in food flavors part I: Dairy products. *Critical Reviews in Food Science & Nutrition*, 3(4), 457-478.

Farkye, N., & Fox, P. F. (1992). Contribution of plasmin to Cheddar cheese ripening: effect of added plasmin. *Journal of Dairy Research*, 59(2), 209-216.

Fernandez-Garcia, E., Lopez-Fandiño, R., Alonso, L., & Ramos, M. (1994). The use of lipolytic and proteolytic enzymes in the manufacture of Manchego type cheese from ovine and bovine milk. *Journal of Dairy Science*, 77(8), 2139-2149.

Fraga, J. L., Penha, A. C., Pereira, D. S., Silva, K. A., Akil, E., Torres, A. G., & Amaral, P. F. (2018). Use of Yarrowia lipolytica Lipase immobilized in cell debris for the production of lipolyzed milk fat (LMF). *International Journal of Molecular Sciences*, 19(11), 3413.

Gandhi, N. N. (1997). Applications of lipase. *Journal of the American Oil Chemists' Society*, 74(6), 621-634.

Guentert, M. (2007). The flavour and fragrance industry—past, present, and future. In *Flavours and Fragrances* (pp. 1-14). Springer, Berlin, Heidelberg.

Hassan, F. A., El-Gawad, A., Mona, A. M., & Enab, A. K. (2012). Flavour compounds in cheese. *International Journal of Academic Research*, 4(5).

https://www.fssai.gov.in/.../Direction_Operationalization_Milk_Standards_04_08_2017.

Ismail, B., & Nielsen, S. S. (2010). Invited review: plasmin protease in milk: current knowledge and relevance to dairy industry. *Journal of Dairy Science*, *93*(11), 4999-5009.

Jaeger,K.E., & Reetz,M.T. (1998). Microbial lipases form versatile tools for biotechnology. *Trends in Biotechnology*, *16*(9), 396-403.

Jensen, R. G. (2002). The composition of bovine milk lipids: January 1995 to December 2000. *Journal of dairy science*, *85*(2), 295-350.

Jooyandeh, H., Amarjeet, K., & Minhas, K. S. (2009). Lipases in dairy industry: a review. *Journal of Food Science and Technology (Mysore)*, *46*(3), 181-189.

Kaminogawa, S., Yamauchi, K., & Tsugo, T. (1969). Properties of milk protease concentrated from acid-precipitated casein. *Japanese Journal of Zootechnical Science*, *40*, 559-565.

Kitchen, B. J. (1971). Bovine milk esterases. *Journal of Dairy Research*, *38*(2), 171-177.

Kontkanen, H., Rokka, S., Kemppinen, A., Miettinen, H., Hellström, J., Kruus, K., & Korhonen, H. (2011). Enzymatic and physical modification of milk fat: A review. *International Dairy Journal*, *21*(1), 3-13.

Kuddus, M. (2019). Introduction to Food Enzymes. In *Enzymes in Food Biotechnology* (pp. 1-18). Academic Press.

Kumar, D. S., & Ray, S. (2014). Fungal lipase production by solid state fermentation-an overview. *Journal of Analytical and Bioanalytical Techniques*, *6*(230), 1-10.

Nunez, M. (2016). Enzymes Exogenous to Milk in Dairy Technology: Proteinases.

Omar, K. A., Gounga, M. E., Liu, R., Mlyuka, E., & Wang, X. (2016). Effects of microbial lipases on hydrolyzed milk fat at different time intervals in flavour development and oxidative stability. *Journal of Food Science and Technology*, *53*(2), 1035-1046.

Qureshi, M. A., Khare, A. K., Pervez, A., & Uprit, S. (2015). Enzymes used in dairy industries. *Int J Appl Res*, *1*(10), 523-527.

Wilkinson M.G., Kilcawley, K.N. (2003). Enzyme modified cheese. In: *Encyclopedia of Dairy Science. Roginski H, Fuquay JW, Fox PF (eds), Academic Press, UK*, p 434-438

Wilkinson, M. G., & Kilcawley, K. N. (2005). Mechanisms of incorporation and release of enzymes into cheese during ripening. *International Dairy Journal*, *15*(6-9), 817-830.

9

Applications of Modified Starch in Dairy and Food Products

***Chandni Dularia*[1] *and Rahul Thory*[2]**

[1]Dairy Technology Division, ICAR-National Dairy Research Institute, Karnal, Haryana, India
[2]School of Bioengineering and Food Technology, Shoolini University, Solan Himachal Pradesh, India

Abstract

Modified starch is very popular and has been used for a long time due to its wide applications in the dairy and food industry. Native starch produces a weak body, rubber-like paste during heating, and undesirable gels during cooling. Hence, to increase starch characteristics like solubility in water, swelling power capacity during cooking, retrogradation tendency, water binding ability, gelling ability, improved structure, and viscosity compared to its native form, modification of starch is done. This chapter deals with the definition and methods or techniques for modifying starches such as physical, chemical, and enzymatic methods. Recent studies on the application of modified starches for different dairy and food products such as bread making, resistant starch muffins, slowly digestible cookies, battered foods or crispy snacks, low-fat & salad mayonnaise, edible packaging/biodegradable package, low-fat yogurt, low-fat cheese, and starch-based dairy dessert have also been discussed. With the rise in consumer's expectations regarding the knowledge about healthy products, the growing population is becoming health conscious. Therefore, the use of modified starch will increase in the dairy and food sector with the introduction of enzyme modification technology as a new field in which the modification of starches is done genetically which can substitute or replace the existing chemical and physical modification methods in the near future.

Introduction

Starch is the most abundant polysaccharide carbohydrate reserve which is available in different parts of plants such as roots, stem, leaves, seeds, flowers, and fruits. It is considered an excellent source of energy and plants utilizes carbon from it for their metabolic activities (Smith, 2001). It is composed of glucose units linked together by glycosidic bonds to form amylose and amylopectin polymeric chains (Abbas *et al*., 2010). The linear chain of amylose comprises of anhydroglucose units linked by α-1, 4 glycosidic bonds. The degree of polymerization is ranged between 100-10000 and molecular weights from 10^4-10^6 (Rapaille and Vanhemelrijck, 1997). Linear chains of glucose units in amylopectin are linked by α-1, 4 glycosidic bonds. It is highly branched at α-1, 6 positions composed of small glucose chains at an interval of 20-26 monomer units. The degree of polymerization is greater than 50000 and molecular weights of 10^7 or more (Durrani and Donald, 1995; Rapaille and Vanhemelrijck, 1997). Various sources of starch are roots (30-70%), tuber (65-85%), legumes (25-50%), cereals (40-90%), and unripened/immature fruits *e.g.* mangos and banana (approx. 70%) (Santana and Meireles, 2014).

Native starches produce a cohesive texture, rubber-like paste when treated at high temperature while during cooling it forms a weak body and undesirable gels. There are some other problems also related to starch properties like water-insoluble at room temperature, high resistivity to enzymatic hydrolysis that leads to a lack of functional properties, and inertness. Therefore, their application is limited in the dairy and food industries (Adzahan, 2002; Singh *et al*., 2007). To improve the behavioral characteristics or properties like texture, solubility, tolerance to the heating temperature modification of starches are carried out which will help in expanding its usefulness in dairy and food product industries as compared to the native starches. Such types of native starch after modification are known to be modified starch (Sweedman *et al*., 2013). Modification of native starch results in the formation of different starch derivatives which are utilized at an extensive level in the food and dairy industry as an additive like stabilizer, thickener, and also provides good textural attributes (Singh *et al*., 2010).

In 2016, the market size of modified starch globally valued at USD 9.36 billion that increased up to USD 9.93 in 2017 (Markets and Markets, 2019). It is expected that the market of modified starch will rise at a CAGR of 5.7% from 2017 to 2025. With an increase in the demands of convenience food and other dairy products, it is estimated that its market will grow globally in the future. One of the leading markets for production, consumption, and end-use application in industries of starch is the United States (Grand View Research, 2019).

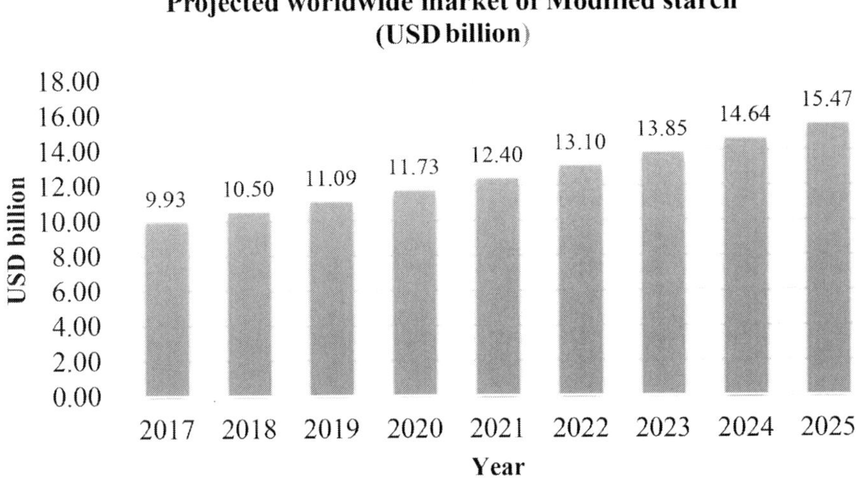

Fig. 9.1: The projected worldwide market of Modified starch at CAGR of 5.7% (USD billion) (*Source*: Grand View Research, 2019)

Methods of Starch Modification

Based on desired characteristics and applications there are various methods adopted to produce modified starches. Different techniques are adopted to change the structural and physicochemical characteristics of starch polymer that helps in making it more flexible and also add value to the food & dairy applications (Lopez *et al.*, 2010). There are three types of methods involved in starch alteration/modification namely, physical, chemical, and enzymatic methods (Yadav *et al.*, 2013).

Physical Modification

For physical modification, starch is modified using heat and moisture (Singh *et al.*, 2007). By physical modification, the properties of starch such as water solubility are improved as well as it also decreases the starch granule size. This process is very cheap, safe, and easy to perform as it adopts various combinations of shear, pressure, moisture, temperature, and irradiation. It is preferred more for human consumption as there is no requirement of the chemical during its production (Ashogbon and Akintayo, 2014). There are different types of physical modifications that are discussed below briefly:

Pre-Gelatinized Starch (PGS)

Cooked starch which is undergone partial gelatinization and further dried is known as pre-gelatinized starch. There are different methods for drying the pre-gelatinized starch such as spray drying, drum drying, and extrusion. During physical modification, granular fragmentation occurs along with loss of birefringence property due to the destruction of the granulated structure of native starch. Different properties such as cold-water dispersion, swelling capacity, and solubility are improved by this method. Based on drying conditions, cooking conditions, and source of starch, the functional properties of PGS are dependent (Ashogbon and Akintayo, 2014). PGS acts as thickeners because of its ability to form pastes and cold-water solubility in several products *e.g.* desserts, soups, and baby foods, *etc.* (Majzoobi *et al.*, 2011).

Hydrothermal Modification

In the hydrothermal modification of starch, conversion of amorphous to a semi-crystalline region takes place due to which there is a change in the physical as well as chemical properties of starch with no destruction in its granule structure (Collado and Corke, 1999; Zavareze and Dias, 2011). Hydrothermal modifications are divided into annealing and hydrothermal (moisture and heat) treatment. Both the treatments cause physical changes with no gelatinization process or starch granule destruction concerning shape, size, or birefringence only by using heat/moisture in a controlled application (Stute, 1992).

Annealing

Starch is modified using the process of annealing in which in the presence of water (40-80%, w/w), heat treatment (25-80 °C) is given that is more than the glass transition temperature and less than the gelatinization temperature with controlled time (hours to days). This process is mild compared to other treatments and no chemical reagents are used in it (Yao *et al.*, 2018). There is no effect caused to the starch granule size and shape. But there may be alterations in the physicochemical properties such as solubility, gelatinization, hydrolysis rate, swelling factor, viscosity, and crystallinity (Tester and Debon, 2000; Yao *et al.*, 2018).

This modification helps in improving the molecular movement and in presence of water, the physical restructuring of the starch granule also occurs (Tester and Debon, 2000). Water acts as a plasticizer for the starch granule, therefore, during the hydration process, it leads to the transformation of starch from glassy to a stable state. Hydration also causes movement of the amorphous regions to crystalline state in starch structure. With these alterations in the crystalline and amorphous regions, radial and tangential movements occur along with the rise in the chain interaction in the crystalline region due to the physicochemical modifications (Chen *et al.*, 2014). The term annealing can only be applied in starch if the temperature during the process does not reach the temperature of gelatinization or when the gelatinization doesn't occur (Tester and Debon, 2000).

Hydrothermal Treatment

In hydrothermal treatment (HMT) the starch is modified in the presence of a controlled quantity of water level (10-30%, w/w) and high heat treatment (90-120 °C) is given for a period of 15 minutes to 16 hours (Maache-Rezzoug *et al.*, 2008; Chung *et al.*, 2009). With the variations in the variety of starch sources and amylose content, there are changes caused by the HMT process in the structure and properties of starch. For example, as compared to cereal or legume starches, the tuber starch is very much sensitive to the HMT process. Hence, they are easily modified in terms of their structure and properties (Hoove and Vasanthan, 1993; Jacobs and Delcour, 1998; Gunaratne and Hoover, 2002).

The hydrothermal treatment causes various effects on the physicochemical and morphological attributes of starch particles such as alteration in the gelatinization, pasting properties, structure crystallinity, swelling capacity, and retrogradation (Hoover, 2010; Hormdok and Noomhorm, 2007; Jyothi *et al.*, 2010). Based on the source of starch, composition, and association of amylose and amylopectin, the changes in the physicochemical and structure of starch are produced during HMT. By such modifications, the altered or modified starch becomes prone to enzymatic and chemical modifications such as acid hydrolysis (Zavareze and Dias, 2011).

Non-thermal Modification

Non-thermal modification treatments were familiarized so that the loss of important vitamins and nutrients caused by traditional treatments can be prevented. Non-thermal treatments help in preserving the organoleptic properties of food and also inhibit the attack of spores and pathogenic microorganisms. There are various types of non-thermal techniques such as ultrasound, high-pressure, and electric pulses (Anderson and Guraya, 2006; Mollekopf *et al.*, 2011; Hodsagi *et al.*, 2012; Brasoveanu and Nemtanu, 2014).

The pressure range used in high-pressure technology is from 400-900 MPa. This technology is used for constraining the swelling capacity that results in the decline of paste viscosity. Atmospheric argon plasma tech nology is one another technology used for starch granule alteration or modification in which the pressure used is very less than the atmospheric pressure (vacuum pressures) (Deeyai *et al.*, 2013; Wongsagonsup *et al.*, 2014). Different types of active ionic species such as excited atoms, protons, and electrons are present in the ionized gas that is plasma (Bogaerts *et al.*, 2002). Several other types of gases are used in plasma state for this technology like oxygen, hydrogen, ethylene, air, methane, ammonia, or argon. This technology alters the starch attributes such as hygroscopicity, oxidation, and degree of polymerization (Wongsagonsup *et al.*, 2014).

Microwave is one another type of starch modification technique in which different mechanisms are interrelated like irradiation, starch characteristics, *etc*. The dielectric properties of starch in the irradiation method is dependent on the moisture and temperature (Braşoveanu and Nemţanu, 2014). The alteration in starch granule by microwave technique influences characteristics of starch like change in swelling power, gelatinization temperature, enthalpies, rheological features, and solubility (Iida *et al.*, 2008; Yu *et al.*, 2013; Zuo *et al.*, 2012). Morphological and crystallinity changes in starch granules are dependent on the type of source and moisture content of starch during microwave treatment (Brasoveanu and Nemtanu, 2014).

Ultrasound is a physical type of method for the starch modification that is applied to gelatinized starch and starch suspension (Iida *et al.*, 2008; Yu *et al.*, 2013; Zuo *et al.*, 2012). This treatment doesn't affect the starch shape and size but primarily causes changes in the amorphous region and also the surface of starch becomes porous. Various attributes of starch are also altered like viscosity, solubility, and swelling power (Luo *et al.*, 2008). This treatment depends on frequency, temperature, process time, sound, and suspension properties of starch (Zuo *et al.*, 2009).

Other Physical Modification: Grinding and Extrusion

Grinding and extrusion are the two main large-scale processes that cause maximum starch granule damage. Shear forces are used in both processes. During grinding, when the shear force is applied, it compresses the starch granule that results in cracks in the starch surface and causes structure damage (Grant, 1998; Liu *et al.*, 2011).

Similarly, extrusion is done along with high temperature and short-time treatment. During this process, the starch granules are exposed to the mechanical shearing action at a low moisture level which helps in increasing the gelatinization temperature. Increase in gelatinization temperature, variations in the molecular extension, and association of starch *e.g.* amylose-lipid complex structure. The resistant starch content is reduced and starch digestibility is improved by this technique (Martinez *et al.*, 2014).

Chemical Modification

During chemical modification, the changes take place due to the addition of any functional group or new chemical in the starch due to which the physicochemical attributes of starch are altered without any change in the structure and size of the starch molecule. There are three major sites in the starch molecule for the chemical modifications which take place at three reactive hydroxyl groups present at each glucose unit in amylose and amylopectin chain. Various physical behavior, such as salting, gelatinization, and retrogradation is changed that helps in maintaining balance in the intermolecular and intramolecular binding of starch granules during chemical modifications (Hernandez, 2018; Korma *et al.,* 2016). There are various methods for chemical modification that are discussed as follows:

Cationization

Cationization is a method in which starch is treated with different cationic molecules. The starch molecules that contain tertiary or quaternary phosphates, ammonium, amino, imino, and sulphuric groups. Native starch contains free hydroxyl groups that are altered by the cationic monomers *e.g.* 3-cholor-2-hydroxypropyl trimethyl ammonium chloride (CTA) or 2, 3-epoxypropyl trimethyl ammonium chloride (ETMAC) in the wet or dry process (Zhang, 2001; Singh *et al.*, 2010). There are three types of cationization methods i.e. dry, wet, and semi-dry cationization. In dry cationization, citric acid is dry heated to convert into anhydride form. During extrusion, the cationic molecules are sprinkled on dried starch in the absence of liquid (Liu *et al.*, 2015; Neelam *et al.*, 2012). Wet cationization occurs in the presence of a liquid phase in which the heterogenous and homogenous reactions between starch and cationic molecules takes place. While in the semi-dry cationization method, the cationic molecules and starch are mixed before the thermal treatment (Liu *et al.*, 2015).

During the cationization process, a high degree of substitution causes changes in the physicochemical attributes of the starch and granular structure. In different sources of starch, this process causes a decline in the pasting temperature while progress in the viscosity peak that results in several changes in starches. This process is very popular in the textile industries (Hubbe, 2006).

Cross-Linking

Cross-linking is a method in which the formation of inter and intramolecular bridges occurs between the linear or branched chains of polymers. Cross-linking is also known as cross-ligation (Korma *et al.*, 2016; Singh *et al.*, 2007).

During this method, hydrogen bonds are substituted by permanent, stronger covalent bonds existing between the starch chains. The most commonly found cross-linked starch is adipate or distarch phosphate (Singh *et al.*, 2010). A three-dimensional network is formed which increases the rigidity of the polymer. Reagents used in crosslinking are sodium tripolyphosphate (STPP), phosphoryl chloride (PDCl3), sodium trimetaphosphate (STMP), and epichlorohydrin (ECH) (Woo and Seib, 2002).

Final product properties such as swelling power and starch paste clarity are dependent on the methods, parameter considered for crosslinking modification, and source of starch. Swelling power and starch paste clarity attributes are interrelated with each other. With the decline in the swelling power, there will be a decline in the starch paste clarity (Kaur *et al.*, 2006; Koo *et al.*, 2010). Moisture, proteins, and lipids are also reduced with the rise in the degree of the crosslinking process. These alterations are caused by various crosslinking agents in different proportions (Carmona-Garcia *et al.*, 2009). Crosslinked starch is used as a thickener and stabilizing agent in frozen foods as it provides clarity and resists the retrogradation process (Lopez *et al.*, 2010).

Acetylation

During the preparation of acetylated starch, the free hydroxyl groups existing in the branched chains of polymeric starch molecules are reacted with acetylated groups (CH_3CO) that produce starch ester (Sweedman *et al.*, 2013). The resistance of bonds between the starch molecules decreases when acetyl groups are introduced (Berski *et al.*, 2011). The crystallinity or retrogradation process of starch granules is hindered after acetylation treatment (Thirumdas *et al.*, 2017). After modification of native starch using acetylation, the swelling power and solubility are improved compared to the native starch (Berski *et al.*, 2011).

Acid Hydrolysis

In acid hydrolysis, starch is treated with acidic solutions (mostly used are H_2SO_4 or HCl) below their T_g (gelatinization temperature) for different time intervals. The α-1, 4 and α-1, 6 linkages or bonds are broken down into short polymeric chains. The degree of hydrolysis is analyzed by the viscosity of cooked modified starch. The starch paste attained after completion of the treatment is neutralized by washing until the pH becomes neutral. The starch slurry is further dried to convert into powder form. The structure and functional properties of acid hydrolyzed starch is also altered after the treatment. The final molecular mass of the starch granules declines with an increase in its crystalline structure (Zuo *et al.*, 2014; Amaya-Llano *et al.*, 2008; Hoover, 2000).

After the completion of acid hydrolysis, crystallinity property in starch is increased while there is a decline in the molecular mass of starch particles (Zuo *et al.*, 2014). The level of amylose is also reduced which leads to an increase in the pasting temperature and gelatinization enthalpies of starch granules (Lawal, 2004). When a diluted form of acid is used it leads to improvement in the gel consistency while the viscosity of the starch paste is reduced because of the depolymerization process (Pérez and Bertoft, 2010; Ulbrich *et al.*, 2014).

Oxidation

Oxidized starch is a starch that is altered due to the introduction of a functional group such as carbonyl or carboxyl groups in the starch molecule. This helps in the depolymerization of the starch molecule (Kuakpetoon and Wang, 2001). Some conditions like pH and temperature are maintained during oxidation treatment. Potassium permanganate, sodium hypochlorite, chromic acid, per-acetic acid, hydrogen peroxide, and nitrogen dioxide are the reactive oxidants used in the modification of starch by oxidation method (Sandhu *et al.*, 2008; Sánchez-Rivera *et al.*, 2005; Wang and Wang, 2003).

Dual Modifications

Different physical and chemical methods are combined or two chemical methods can be used together for the modification of starch granules *e.g.* acetylation combined with microwave (chemical and physical); acetylation along with oxidation (a combination of chemical methods) (Ashogbon and Akintayo, 2014; Adebowale and Lawal, 2002).

Enzymatic Modification

Amylase enzymes (α-amylase and β-amylase) are used for the starch modification that helps in developing derivative with good adhesion property. It is mostly used in food coating with a colorant and in bakery industries (Park *et al.*, 2018).

Application of Modified Starch in Dairy and Food Products

Dairy Products

Modified starches are utilized in different dairy products. It gives variable effects such as enhanced mouthfeel, stability, viscosity and cuttability. In yogurt and sour creams, modified starches are used to enhance thickness and control the syneresis process.

Low-fat Yogurt

Studies on low-fat yogurt reveal that fat used in the yogurt could be replaced by using modified starch. Modified waxy maize starch (MWMS) added at 1.5g/kg milk for the preparation of low-fat yogurt showed a compact texture with a reduced amount of syneresis process and exhibited textural properties similar to that full-fat yogurt (Abbas *et al.*, 2017).

It was considered that the creaminess of low-fat yogurt can be improved by the application of amylomaltase-treated starch (ATS). ATS is four times effective as maltodextrin and acts as a creaminess enhancer. The perception of creaminess can be increased from 1.5% in low-fat yogurt to 5% in full-fat yogurt with the addition of ATS in small amounts. The protein network of yogurt is very dominant that encapsulates or encloses the ATS domains. During consumption of yogurt with added ATS, these ATS domains are melted in the mouth by which its creaminess is perceived. This perception arises by the mutual effect of physical melting and hydrolysis by the action salivary amylase enzyme existing in the saliva (Alting *et al.*, 2009).

Low-fat Cheese

Kashar cheese or Turkish traditional cheese was produced using two protein-based fat substitutes or replacer i.e. Simplesse ®D-100 (1.0% w/w) and Dairy-Lo™ (1% w/w) with a carbohydrate-based fat substitute or replacer i.e. Raftiline ®HP. During 90 days of storage, it was observed that springiness, hardness, chewiness, and gumminess deteriorated with the use of fat substitute or replacer while cohesiveness property improved. Cheese meltability was increased slightly with the use of a carbohydrate-based fat substitute or replacer, Raftiline ®HP. This suggested that Simplesse ®D-100 and Raftiline ®HP are responsible for the improvement in the textural and sensorial characteristics of low-fat fresh Kashar cheese (Koca and Metin, 2004).

Many other fat replacers or substitute can also be used as in cheeses for reducing fat such as lecithin and tapioca starch. When fat is reduced, the moisture, hardness, and protein content levels are increased. Cheeses made without any fat mimetic that contained 0.2% lecithin, 1% modified tapioca starch, and blend of 0.5% tapioca starch and 0.1% lecithin. Fat 9-16% was used for manufacturing low-fat Feta cheeses in which before analysis, the bovine milk (1.6-2.2% fat) was ripened for 45 days. Fat and fat mimetics levels didn't affect the protein, moisture, hardness, and yield of the prepared cheeses. Reduced-fat cheeses prepared using modified tapioca starch had the least protein (13.5%), higher moisture (67.6%), and higher hardness. With a decrease in the level of fat, the protein started to aggregate more. While a mixture of modified tapioca and lecithin used in the preparation of reduced-fat and low-fat feta cheese improved the flavor, texture, and overall acceptability (Sipahioglu *et al.,* 2000).

Starch-based Dairy Dessert

Starch-based dairy desserts are also known as pudding which is formulated using milk, starch/hydrocolloids, coloring agents, flavoring agents, and sugar. This is very popular among all groups of consumers from young to old aged people (Tarrega and Costell, 2006). Different types of plants are used for the production of inulin that can be added to the starch-based dairy dessert. They are non-digestible polysaccharides that are linked by β-(2-1) fructose residues with a terminal glucose residue unit (Izzo and Niness, 2001; Flamm *et al*., 2001). They are dietary fiber as they are resistant to the human digestive enzymatic hydrolysis (Flamm *et al.,* 2001).

Waxy corn starch was added at the rate of 2.5, 3.25, and 4% along with inulin for preparing fat-free dairy desserts and compared with full-fat milk samples. The rheological flow behavior showed that it possessed thixotropic and shear-thinning flow behavior. For obtaining optimum rheological flow behavior, modified starch is added on which the addition of inulin is dependent. For the desirable texture, hydroxypropylated starch from waxy corn along with carrageenan could be used (Tarrega and Costell, 2006).

Bakery

Bakery products are also comprised of modified starches that help in providing different properties such as, good cuttability, stability during baking, storage stability (no water separation after 48 hours), fine structure, short texture, direct setting, and freeze-thaw stability.

Bread Making

For manufacturing the bread, starch plays an important role in giving textural attributes in dough making. Some unwanted properties of native starch that affect the texture and quality are diminished by the use of modified starches during bread-making.

Starch functional properties can be obtained in the bread-making by the utilization of waxy wheat flour (WWF) and high-amylose wheat flour (HAWF). During seven days of storage and also after reheating, the breadcrumbs continued to have a soft texture when they are made by the use of WWF compared to HAWF and non-waxy wheat flour. While with the rise in reheating causes an increase in the firmness in the case of HAWF and non- waxy wheat flour in comparison with the pre-heated breadcrumbs. This suggests that waxy wheat flour used for making bread had more glutinous, viscous, and soft attributes of breadcrumbs (Van Hung *et al.,* 2006).

Bread crumb was dry in texture and lower peak viscosity with a lesser breakdown on the amylogram was observed when phosphorylated cross-linked tapioca starch was used for making the bread. When flour was replaced by native, hydroxypropylated, and acetylated tapioca starch, there was an increase in the stickiness property in the bread and higher peak viscosity with a large breakdown on the amylogram (Miyazaki *et al.* 2005, 2006).

Slowly Digestible Cookies

Slowly digestible cookies prepared using resistant-starch rich powder (RSRP) attained from autoclave-treated lintnerized banana starch showed that the best formulation was wheat flour: RSRP (15:85). Based on the prediction of hydrolysis index (HI), wheat flour: RSRP cookies (60.71 ± 2.28) showed a lesser value of HI compared to control cookies (80.54 ± 2.64). Also, the prediction glycemic index for wheat flour: RSRP cookies had 60.53 while compared with control cookies had 77.62. This suggests that in bakery products RSRP from banana starch can be utilized that will help in the slow release of carbohydrate. It will also help in developing products that have low caloric and glycemic index (Aparicio-Saguilan *et al.*, 2007).

Resistant Starch Muffins

Resistant starch obtained from native maize was made to substitute the wheat flour that displayed a reduction in the height, volume, and area of gas bubbles in the muffins. The structural elements given by the wheat flour were also declined when more than 10% of resistant starch was used as a substitute (Baixauli *et al.*, 2008a).

Further study on the acceptability of consumers was conducted in two sessions in which plain muffins, resistant starch muffins, and lastly whole meal muffins from the local market were presented before the consumers. The evaluation was responded based on "appearance", "texture", "flavor" and "overall acceptability". The first session dealt with the evaluation of muffins without any knowledge of nutritional information. In the second session, an evaluation was done in which the information regarding health effects and its benefits were given. In the first session, whole meal muffins scored lowest but in later sessions due to its high fiber levels, the scores were increased which indicates that nutritional information and health benefits play an important part in consumer perception. While in the case of resistant starch muffins, the increment in the scores was lower even after the knowledge given about its fiber content similar to the whole meal muffin. The appearance may be one of the reasons for its lower scores compared to whole meal muffin (Baixauli *et al.,* 2008b).

Battered Food/Crispy Snacks

For the improvement in the appearance and palatability of deep-fat fried products, batters are prepared. The important quality of most of the battered food is the crispiness of the product. These battered foods contain a considerable amount of fat in it. Consumption of deep-fat fried products with high fat/oil content causes various diseases like cardiovascular attack and obesity. So, to minimize such high fat/oil content in these products modified starches are used (Altunakar *et al.*, 2004; Rimac-Brncic *et al.*, 2004).

For the preparation of fried battered chicken, wheat flour (10% w/w) was replaced by 2 modified starches namely, crispcoat® (a blend of high amylose corn starch and tapioca dextrin) crispfilm® (modified high amylose corn starch) in the batter formula.

For crispcoat® and crispfilm® batters, moisture content, amylose content, oil content, peak viscosity and batter pick-up were 39.39%, 29.87%, 30.50%, 1331.00 cP, 29.38% and 25.25%, 31.87%, 20.29%, 1657.67 cP, 32.93%, respectively. Oil absorption in the fried battered chicken was found lowest prepared using crispfilm® modified starch that suggests better quality of the product (Vongsawasdi *et al.*, 2008).

Different starch types like corn, waxy maize, amylomaize, pre-gelatinized tapioca were used that affect the quality attributes such as moisture content, color, oil content, texture, volume, cooking yield, porosity, and coating pick-up of the product. Deep-fat fried chicken nuggets were prepared using the batter coating (equivalent amount of corn and wheat flour, 5.0% starch, 0.5% leavening agent, and 1.0% salt) on the breast portion. At the last step of frying, crispiness was improved with an increase in the starch content. While with the rise in the frying time there was a reduction in the moisture content. Other starch types were also used in place of corn which indicated that the best results were obtained using pre-gelatinized starch that had high moisture content, volume, better coating pick-up, and least oil content in the deep-fat fried chicken nuggets (Altunakar *et al.*, 2004).

Low-fat Mayonnaise

Mayonnaise is an oil-in-water (O/W) type of emulsion. It is semi-solid and prepared using the proper blending of oil (70-80%), vinegar, spices, and egg yolk. Egg yolk is the key ingredient and acts as an emulsifying agent in mayonnaise that provides stability to the product. Due to high fat and cholesterol levels, various health-related diseases like obesity and cardiovascular-related diseases occur. Hence, to prevent such condition fat is substituted by modified starch (Mirzanajafi-Zanjani *et al.,* 2019).

Gluten can be used as a fat replacer or substitute in mayonnaise. Gluten based mayonnaise was compared with egg-yolk based mayonnaise. The results indicated that wheat gluten was added the optimum fat percentage replaced at 1.0% showed identical textural (smoothness, sliminess, and creaminess) and sensorial properties, very similar fat size droplet distribution compared to the egg-yolk based mayonnaise (Liu *et al.*, 2018).

Oat dextrin was utilized as a fat substitute that made fat granules smaller in size, uniformly distributed, and symmetric in size when the optimum fat percentage replaced was 27.9% (Shen *et al.*, 2011).

No differences were found in the viscosity, yield stress, and flow behavior index between two low-fat containing mayonnaise (comprised of xanthan gum + 10 g kg^{-1} guar gum and citrus fiber + 5 g kg^{-1} guar gum) compared to control mayonnaise (full-fat mayonnaise). Sensorial scores also showed that there were no differences among low-fat mayonnaise comprised of xanthan gum + 10 g kg^{-1} guar gum and control mayonnaise (Su *et al.,* 2010).

Salad Mayonnaise

Modified starch can act as a gelling agent and provides stability to the low-fat salad dressings/mayonnaise at high-shear emulsion. Scanning electron microscopy study reveals that the oil droplets form aggregates that are smaller in size and uniformly distributed in a network of carbohydrates. The stability is higher for the low-fat salad mayonnaise that uses modified starch during preparation when compared to the control full-fat mayonnaise or full-fat salad dressing. Strong gels are formed which are responsible for the high stability in the product even at high shear rates (Depree and Savage, 2001).

Edible Packaging Films/Edible Films/Biodegradable Films

Due to environmental issues, various health-related concerns, and unsatisfactory mechanical and barrier properties of packaging material have led to the demand for biodegradable film or edible films. These films have different functions such as increasing the senescence and maturity period of perishable fruits and vegetables, prevents the microbial attack and maintains post-harvest quality (Jimenez *et al.,* 2013). Different environment-friendly biopolymers are used for the preparation of these films such as proteins, starch, lipids, and polysaccharides (Di Pierro *et al.*, 2007, 2011; Dularia *et al.*, 2019).

For preparing edible films starch along with chitosan are used widely for preserving food. The casting method was applied for film preparation using chitosan (CT), acetylated (AS), waxy (WS), and oxidized (OS) corn starches and their mixtures. Among films prepared using individual components, CT starch films presented good barrier and mechanical properties. While among the mixtures, CT-OS film was having the lowest water content, thickness, solubility, hardness, surface roughness, and water vapor transmission rate. Based on the method adopted for modifying the starch, the interaction with chitosan leads to a change in the film properties (Escamilla-Garcia *et al.*, 2017).

Conclusion

Starch is known for its wide application in many foods and dairy products and other non-food industries due to its nutritional and functional attributes. The use of native starch in industries is very less because of the problem of less solubility in water. Therefore, to overcome such problems different modification methods are used. These modification methods of starch have led to increasing the starch solubility, water-binding ability, gelling ability, improved structure, viscosity, after cooking swelling capacity, retrogradation tendency quality.

Modified starch is now becoming very popular among the food and dairy industries. These modified starches can be used for manufacturing different food group category products in which they can act as texture improver, fat replacer or substitute, high nutritional product, edible package material, *etc.* Other than this, they also act as a thickening agent, binding agent, water-binding ability, gelling ability, emulsifier, stabilizer, drying aids, *etc.*

As the consumers are now becoming aware of their health, therefore the demands for healthy foods will be increasing day by day. Enzyme modification technique is the new field in which the modification of starches is done genetically which can substitute or replace the existing chemical and physical modification methods in the near future.

References

Abbas, K. A., El-Garhi, H. M., & Hamdy, S. M. (2017). The Influence of Modified Waxy Maize Starch on the Quality of Low-Fat Yogurt. *Egyptian Journal of Food Science*. 45*(1)*, 171-177.

Abbas, K. A., Khalil, S. K., & Hussin, A. S. M. (2010). Modified starches and their usages in selected food products: a review study. *Journal of Agricultural Science*, *2*(2), 90-100.

Adebowale, K. O., and Lawal, O. S. (2002). Effect of annealing and heat moisture conditioning on the physicochemical characteristics of Bambarra groundnut (*Voandzeia subterranea*) starch. *Food/Nahrung*, *46*(5), 311-316.

Adzahan, N. M. (2002). Modification on wheat, sago and tapioca starches by irradiation and its effect on the physical properties of fish cracker (keropok)(Master's thesis). *Food Technology. Selangor, University of Putra Malaysia.*

Alting, A. C., Van de Velde, F., Kanning, M. W., Burgering, M., Mulleners, L., Sein, A., & Buwalda, P. (2009). Improved creaminess of low-fat yoghurt: The impact of amylomaltase-treated starch domains. *Food Hydrocolloids*, *23*(3), 980-987.

Altunakar, B., Sahin, S., & Sumnu, G. (2004). Functionality of batters containing different starch types for deep-fat frying of chicken nuggets. *European Food Research and Technology*, *218*(4), 318-322.

Amaya-Llano, S. L., Martinez-Alegria, A. L., Zazueta-Morales, J. J., & Martinez-Bustos, F. (2008). Acid thinned jicama and maize starches as fat substitute in stirred yogurt. *LWT-Food Science and Technology*, *41*(7), 1274-1281.

Anderson, A. K., & Guraya, H. S. (2006). Effects of microwave heat-moisture treatment on properties of waxy and non-waxy rice starches. *Food Chemistry*, *97*(2), 318-323.

Aparicio-Saguilan, A., Sayago-Ayerdi, S. G., Vargas-Torres, A., Tovar, J., Ascencio-Otero, T. E., & Bello-Perez, L. A. (2007). Slowly digestible cookies prepared from resistant starch-rich lintnerized banana starch. *Journal of Food composition and Analysis*, *20*(3-4), 175-181.

Ashogbon, A. O., & Akintayo, E. T. (2014). Recent trend in the physical and chemical modification of starches from different botanical sources: A review. *Starch-Starke*, *66*(1-2), 41-57.

Baixauli, R., Salvador, A., Hough, G., & Fiszman, S. M. (2008b). How information about fibre (traditional and resistant starch) influences consumer acceptance of muffins. *Food Quality and Preference*, *19*(7), 628-635.

Baixauli, R., Sanz, T., Salvador, A., & Fiszman, S. M. (2008a). Muffins with resistant starch: Baking performance in relation to the rheological properties of the batter. *Journal of Cereal Science*, *47*(3), 502-509.

Berski, W., Ptaszek, A., Ptaszek, P., Ziobro, R., Kowalski, G., Grzesik, M., & Achremowicz, B. J. C. P. (2011). Pasting and rheological properties of oat starch and its derivatives. *Carbohydrate Polymers*, *83*(2), 665-671.

Bogaerts, A., Neyts, E., Gijbels, R., & Van der Mullen, J. (2002). Gas discharge plasmas and their applications. *Spectrochimica Acta Part B: Atomic Spectroscopy*, *57*(4), 609-658.

Braşoveanu, M., & Nemţanu, M. R. (2014). Behaviour of starch exposed to microwave radiation treatment. *Starch□Starke*, *66*(1-2), 3-14.

Carmona-Garcia, R., Sanchez-Rivera, M. M., Mendez-Montealvo, G., Garza-Montoya, B., & Bello-Perez, L. A. (2009). Effect of the cross-linked reagent type on some morphological, physicochemical and functional characteristics of banana starch (Musa paradisiaca). *Carbohydrate Polymers*, *76*(1), 117-122.

Chen, X., He, X., & Huang, Q. (2014). Effects of hydrothermal pretreatment on subsequent octenylsuccinic anhydride (OSA) modification of cornstarch. *Carbohydrate Polymers*, *101*, 493-498.

Chung, H. J., Liu, Q., & Hoover, R. (2009). Impact of annealing and heat-moisture treatment on rapidly digestible, slowly digestible and resistant starch levels in native and gelatinized corn, pea and lentil starches. *Carbohydrate Polymers*, *75*(3), 436-447.

Collado, L. S., & Corke, H. (1999). Heat-moisture treatment effects on sweet potato starches differing in amylose content. *Food Chemistry*, *65*(3), 339-346.

Deeyai, P., Suphantharika, M., Wongsagonsup, R., & Dangtip, S. (2013). Characterization of modified tapioca starch in atmospheric argon plasma under diverse humidity by FTIR spectroscopy. *Chinese Physics Letters*, *30*(1), 018103.

Depree, J. A., & Savage, G. P. (2001). Physical and flavour stability of mayonnaise. *Trends in Food Science & Technology*, *12*(5-6), 157-163.

Di Pierro, P., Chico, B., Villalonga, R., Mariniello, L., Masi, P., & Porta, R. (2007). Transglutaminase-catalyzed preparation of chitosan–ovalbumin films. *Enzyme and Microbial Technology*, *40*(3), 437-441.

Di Pierro, P., Sorrentino, A., Mariniello, L., Giosafatto, C. V. L., & Porta, R. (2011). Chitosan/whey protein film as active coating to extend Ricotta cheese shelf-life. *LWT-Food Science and Technology*, *44*(10), 2324-2327.

Dularia, C., Sinhmar, A., Thory, R., Pathera, A. K., & Nain, V. (2019). Development of starch nanoparticles based composite films from non-conventional source-Water chestnut (Trapa bispinosa). *International Journal of Biological Macromolecules*, *136*, 1161-1168.

Durrani, C. M., & Donald, A. M. (1995). Physical characterisation of amylopectin gels. *Polymer Gels and Networks*, *3*(1), 1-27.

Escamilla-Garcia, M., Reyes-Basurto, A., Garcia-Almendarez, B. E., Hernandez-Hernandez, E., Calderon-Dominguez, G., Rossi-Marquez, G., & Regalado-Gonzalez, C. (2017). Modified starch-chitosan edible films: Physicochemical and mechanical characterization. *Coatings*, *7*(12), 224.

Flamm, G., Glinsmann, W., Kritchevsky, D., Prosky, L., & Roberfroid, M. (2001). Inulin and oligofructose as dietary fiber: a review of the evidence. *Critical Reviews in Food Science and Nutrition*, *41*(5), 353-362.

Grand View Research (2019), https://www.grandviewresearch.com/industry-analysis/modified-starch-market Accessed on: 11-08-2019.

Grant, L. A. (1998). Effects of starch isolation, drying, and grinding techniques on its gelatinization and retrogradation properties. *Cereal Chemistry*, *75*(5), 590-594.

Gunaratne, A., & Hoover, R. (2002). Effect of heat–moisture treatment on the structure and physicochemical properties of tuber and root starches. *Carbohydrate Polymers*, *49*(4), 425-437.

Hernandez, A. R. (2018). Chemical Modification of Starch with Synthetic. *Applications of Modified Starches*, *2*, 3-22.

Hodsagi, M., Jambor, A., Juhasz, E., Gergely, S., Gelencser, T., & Salgo, A. (2012). Effects of microwave heating on native and resistant starches. *Acta Alimentaria*, *41*(2), 233-247.

Hoove, R., & Vasanthan, T. (1993). The effect of annealing on the physicochemical properties of wheat, oat, potato and lentil starches. *Journal of Food Biochemistry*, *17*(5), 303-325.

Hoover, R. (2000). Acid-treated starches. *Food Reviews International*, *16*(3), 369-392.

Hoover, R. (2010). The impact of heat-moisture treatment on molecular structures and properties of starches isolated from different botanical sources. *Critical Reviews in Food Science and Nutrition*, *50*(9), 835-847.

Hormdok, R., & Noomhorm, A. (2007). Hydrothermal treatments of rice starch for improvement of rice noodle quality. *LWT-Food science and Technology*, *40*(10), 1723-1731.

Hubbe, M. A. (2006). Bonding between cellulosic fibers in the absence and presence of dry-strength agents–A review. *BioResources*, *1*(2), 281-318.

Iida, Y., Tuziuti, T., Yasui, K., Towata, A., & Kozuka, T. (2008). Control of viscosity in starch and polysaccharide solutions with ultrasound after gelatinization. *Innovative Food Science & Emerging Technologies*, *9*(2), 140-146.

Izzo, M., & Niness, K. (2001). Formulating nutrition bars with inulin and oligofructose. *Cereal Foods World*, *46*(3), 102-106.

Jacobs, H., & Delcour, J. A. (1998). Hydrothermal modifications of granular starch, with retention of the granular structure: A review. *Journal of Agricultural and Food Chemistry*, *46*(8), 2895-2905.

Jiménez, A., Fabra, M. J., Talens, P., & Chiralt, A. (2013). Physical properties and antioxidant capacity of starch–sodium caseinate films containing lipids. *Journal of Food Engineering*, *116*(3), 695-702.

Jyothi, A. N., Sajeev, M. S., & Sreekumar, J. N. (2010). Hydrothermal modifications of tropical tuber starches. 1. Effect of heat□moisture treatment on the physicochemical, rheological and gelatinization characteristics. *Starch□Stärke*, *62*(1), 28-40.

Kaur, L., Singh, J., & Singh, N. (2006). Effect of cross□linking on some properties of potato (*Solanum tuberosum* L.) starches. *Journal of the Science of Food and Agriculture*, *86*(12), 1945-1954.

Koca, N., & Metin, M. (2004). Textural, melting and sensory properties of low-fat fresh kashar cheeses produced by using fat replacers. *International Dairy Journal*, *14*(4), 365-373.

Koo, S. H., Lee, K. Y., & Lee, H. G. (2010). Effect of cross-linking on the physicochemical and physiological properties of corn starch. *Food Hydrocolloids*, *24*(6-7), 619-625.

Korma, S. A., Niazi, S., Ammar, A. F., Zaaboul, F., & Zhang, T. (2016). Chemically modified starch and utilization in food stuffs. *International Journal of Nutrition and Food Sciences*, *5*(4), 264.

Kuakpetoon, D., & Wang, Y. J. (2001). Characterization of different starches oxidized by hypochlorite. *Starch□Stärke*, *53*(5), 211-218.

Lawal, O. S. (2004). Composition, physicochemical properties and retrogradation characteristics of native, oxidised, acetylated and acid-thinned new cocoyam (Xanthosoma sagittifolium) starch. *Food Chemistry*, *87*(2), 205-218.

Liu, J., Yang, R., & Yang, F. (2015). Effect of the starch source on the performance of cationic starches having similar degree of substitution for papermaking using deinked pulp. *BioResources*, *10*(1), 922-931.

Liu, T. Y., Ma, Y., Yu, S. F., Shi, J., & Xue, S. (2011). The effect of ball milling treatment on structure and porosity of maize starch granule. *Innovative Food Science & Emerging Technologies*, *12*(4), 586-593.

Liu, X., Guo, J., Wan, Z. L., Liu, Y. Y., Ruan, Q. J., & Yang, X. Q. (2018). Wheat gluten-stabilized high internal phase emulsions as mayonnaise replacers. *Food Hydrocolloids*, *77*, 168-175.

Lopez, O. V., Zaritzky, N. E., & Garcia, M. A. (2010). Physicochemical characterization of chemically modified corn starches related to rheological behavior, retrogradation and film forming capacity. *Journal of Food Engineering*, *100*(1), 160-168.

Luo, Z., Fu, X., He, X., Luo, F., Gao, Q., & Yu, S. (2008). Effect of ultrasonic treatment on the physicochemical properties of maize starches differing in amylose content. *Starch-Stärke*, *60*(11), 646-653.

Maache-Rezzoug, Z., Zarguili, I., Loisel, C., Queveau, D., & Buleon, A. (2008). Structural modifications and thermal transitions of standard maize starch after DIC hydrothermal treatment. *Carbohydrate Polymers*, *74*(4), 802-812.

Majzoobi, M., Radi, M., Farahnaky, A., Jamalian, J., Tongdang, T., & Mesbahi, G. (2011). Physicochemical properties of pre-gelatinized wheat starch produced by a twin drum drier. *Journal of Agricultural Science and Technology*, 13(2), 193-202.

Markets & Markets (2019), https://www.marketsandmarkets.com/Market-Reports/modified-starch-market-511.html Accessed on: 11-08-2020

Martínez, M. M., Rosell, C. M., & Gomez, M. (2014). Modification of wheat flour functionality and digestibility through different extrusion conditions. *Journal of Food Engineering*, *143*, 74-79.

Mirzanajafi-Zanjani, M., Yousefi, M., & Ehsani, A. (2019). Challenges and approaches for production of a healthy and functional mayonnaise sauce. *Food Science & Nutrition*, *7*(8), 2471-2484.

Miyazaki, M., Maeda, T., & Morita, N. (2005). Gelatinization properties and bread quality of flours substituted with hydroxypropylated, acetylated and phosphorylated cross-linked tapioca starches. *Journal of Applied Glycoscience*, *52*(4), 345-350.

Miyazaki, M., Van Hung, P., Maeda, T., & Morita, N. (2006). Recent advances in application of modified starches for breadmaking. *Trends in Food Science & Technology*, *17*(11), 591-599.

Mollekopf, N., Treppe, K., Fiala, P., & Dixit, O. (2011). Vacuum microwave treatment of potato starch and the resultant modification of properties. *Chemie Ingenieur Technik*, *83*(3), 262-272.

Neelam, K., Vijay, S., & Lalit, S. (2012). Various techniques for the modification of starch and the applications of its derivatives. *International Research Journal of Pharmacy*, *3*(5), 25-31.

Park, S. H., Na, Y., Kim, J., Dal Kang, S., & Park, K. H. (2018). Properties and applications of starch modifying enzymes for use in the baking industry. *Food Science and Biotechnology*, *27*(2), 299-312.

Pérez, S., & Bertoft, E. (2010). The molecular structures of starch components and their contribution to the architecture of starch granules: A comprehensive review. *Starch-Starke*, *62*(8), 389-420.

Rapaille, A., & Vanhemelrijck, J. (1997). Modified starches. In Imeson, A. (Ed.) *Thickening and Gelling Agents for Food* (pp. 199-229). Springer, Boston, MA.

Rimac-Brncic, S., Lelas, V., Rade, D., & Simundic, B. (2004). Decreasing of oil absorption in potato strips during deep fat frying. *Journal of Food Engineering*, *64*(2), 237-241.

Sanchez-Rivera, M. M., Garcia-Suarez, F. J. L., Del Valle, M. V., Gutierrez-Meraz, F., & Bello-Perez, L. A. (2005). Partial characterization of banana starches oxidized by different levels of sodium hypochlorite. *Carbohydrate Polymers*, *62*(1), 50-56.

Sandhu, K. S., Kaur, M., Singh, N., & Lim, S. T. (2008). A comparison of native and oxidized normal and waxy corn starches: Physicochemical, thermal, morphological and pasting properties. *LWT-Food Science and Technology*, *41*(6), 1000-1010.

Santana, A. L., & Meireles, M. A. A. (2014). New starches are the trend for industry applications: a review. *Food and Public Health*, *4*(5), 229-241.

Shen, R., Luo, S., & Dong, J. (2011). Application of oat dextrine for fat substitute in mayonnaise. *Food Chemistry*, *126*(1), 65-71.

Singh, A. V., Nath, L. K., & Singh, A. (2010). Pharmaceutical, food and non-food applications of modified starches: a critical review. *Electronic Journal of Environmental, Agricultural and Food Chemistry*, *9*(7), 1214-1221.

Singh, J., Kaur, L., & McCarthy, O. J. (2007). Factors influencing the physico-chemical, morphological, thermal and rheological properties of some chemically modified starches for food applications—A review. *Food Hydrocolloids*, *21*(1), 1-22.

Sipahioglu, O., Alvarez, V. B., & Solano-Lopez, C. (2000). Structure, physico-chemical and sensory properties of Feta cheese made with tapioca starch and lecithin as fat mimetics. *International Dairy Journal*, *9*(11), 783-789.

Smith, A. M. (2001). The biosynthesis of starch granules. *Biomacromolecules*, *2*(2), 335-341.

Stute, R. (1992). Hydrothermal modification of starches: The difference between annealing and heat/moisture-treatment. *Starch-Starke*, *44*(6), 205-214.

Su, H. P., Lien, C. P., Lee, T. A., & Ho, J. H. (2010). Development of low□fat mayonnaise containing polysaccharide gums as functional ingredients. *Journal of the Science of Food and Agriculture*, *90*(5), 806-812.

Sweedman, M. C., Tizzotti, M. J., Schafer, C., & Gilbert, R. G. (2013). Structure and physicochemical properties of octenyl succinic anhydride modified starches: A review. *Carbohydrate Polymers*, *92*(1), 905-920.

Tarrega, A., & Costell, E. (2006). Effect of inulin addition on rheological and sensory properties of fat-free starch-based dairy desserts. *International Dairy Journal*, *16*(9), 1104-1112.

Tester, R., & Debon, S. (2000). Annealing of starch–a review. *International Journal of Biological Macromolecules*, 27*(1)*, 1-12.

Thirumdas, R., Trimukhe, A., Deshmukh, R. R., & Annapure, U. S. (2017). Functional and rheological properties of cold plasma treated rice starch. *Carbohydrate Polymers*, *157*, 1723-1731.

Ulbrich, M., Natan, C., & Floter, E. (2014). Acid modification of wheat, potato, and pea starch applying gentle conditions—impacts on starch properties. *Starch□Starke*, *66*(9-10), 903-913.

Van Hung, P., Macda, T., & Morita, N. (2006). Waxy and high-amylose wheat starches and flours—characteristics, functionality and application. *Trends in Food Science & Technology*, *17*(8), 448-456.

Vongsawasdi, P., Nopharatana, M., Srisuwatchree, W., Pasukcharoenying, S., & Wongkitcharoen, N. (2008). Using modified starch to decrease the oil absorption in fried battered chicken. *Asian Journal of Food and Agro-Industry*, *1*(03), 174-183.

Wang, Y. J., & Wang, L. (2003). Physicochemical properties of common and waxy corn starches oxidized by different levels of sodium hypochlorite. *Carbohydrate Polymers*, *52*(3), 207-217.

Wongsagonsup, R., Deeyai, P., Chaiwat, W., Horrungsiwat, S., Leejariensuk, K., Suphantharika, M., Fuongfuchat, A., & Dangtip, S. (2014). Modification of tapioca starch by non-chemical route using jet atmospheric argon plasma. *Carbohydrate Polymers*, *102*, 790-798.

Woo, K. S., & Seib, P. A. (2002). Cross□linked resistant starch: Preparation and properties. *Cereal Chemistry*, *79*(6), 819-825.

Yadav, B. S., Guleria, P., & Yadav, R. B. (2013). Hydrothermal modification of Indian water chestnut starch: Influence of heat-moisture treatment and annealing on the physicochemical, gelatinization and pasting characteristics. *LWT-Food Science and Technology*, *53*(1), 211-217.

Yao, T., Sui, Z., & Janaswamy, S. (2018). Annealing. In Sui, Z., and Kong, X. (Eds.) *Physical modifications of starch* (pp. 37-49). Springer, Singapore.

Yu, S., Zhang, Y., Ge, Y., Zhang, Y., Sun, T., Jiao, Y., & Zheng, X. Q. (2013). Effects of ultrasound processing on the thermal and retrogradation properties of nonwaxy rice starch. *Journal of Food Process Engineering*, *36*(6), 793-802.

Zavareze, E. D. R., & Dias, A. R. G. (2011). Impact of heat-moisture treatment and annealing in starches: A review. *Carbohydrate Polymers*, *83*(2), 317-328.

Zhang, L. M. (2001). A review of starches and their derivatives for oilfield applications in China. *Starch□Starke*, *53*(9), 401-407.

Zuo, J. Y., Knoerzer, K., Mawson, R., Kentish, S., & Ashokkumar, M. (2009). The pasting properties of sonicated waxy rice starch suspensions. *Ultrasonics Sonochemistry*, *16*(4), 462-468.

Zuo, Y. Y. J., Hebraud, P., Hemar, Y., & Ashokkumar, M. (2012). Quantification of high-power ultrasound induced damage on potato starch granules using light microscopy. *Ultrasonics Sonochemistry*, *19*(3), 421-426.

Zuo, Y., Gu, J., Tan, H., Qiao, Z., Xie, Y., & Zhang, Y. (2014). The characterization of granule structural changes in acid-thinning starches by new methods and its effect on other properties. *Journal of Adhesion Science and Technology*, *28*(5), 479-489.

10

Applications of Nano Science in Dairy Quality Aspect

Payal Karmakar[1] and Ronit Mandal[2]

[1]*Division of Dairy Chemistry, National Dairy Research Institute Karnal Haryana, India*
[2]*Faculty of Land and Food Systems, University of British Columbia Vancouver-V61 1Z4, British Columbia, Canada*

Abstract

Nano science is one of the important advancements in the field of scientific study. It has brought a revolution, the wave of which has influenced many industries, dairy industry being one of them. It has the potential of substituting several technologies by virtue of its immense potential benefits. With the incorporation of nano science, now, the dairy foods are not only good sources of nutrients but also have excellent functional properties and improved sensory attributes. Noteworthy research work has been carried out regarding the encapsulation and delivery of bioactive compounds, which will have increased absorption and enhanced bioavailability. Packaging material with strengthened mechanical barriers and antimicrobials is another beneficial application of nano science. Nano sensors can help in tracing the quality of the food from farm to fork. Rapid sampling of chemical and biological contaminants, bio-separation of proteins, nano encapsulation of nutraceuticals and smart delivery of nutrients are few other areas of emerging interest. However, the undiscovered risk of nano particles towards human health and environmental safety still raises a concern. This chapter deals with the applications of nano science that has affected the field of dairy and the aspects of its quality.

Introduction

The term nanoscience defines controlling or modifying the shapes and sizes of the materials such that they lie in the range of a nanometre (1 nm = 10^{-9} m) scale, typically 1-100 nm (Chavada *et al.*, 2016). The application of these materials and systems by their suitable designing and production is what is known as nanotechnology. Richard Feynman, in 1959, first discussed the possibility of this advanced technology. However, the term was first used by Norio Taniguchi in 1974 (Chavada *et al.,* 2016). Particles having size reduced to this nanometric range show unique properties which are quite different from those of macro particles of same composition (Ravichandran and Sasi, 2006).

The world has been witnessing skyrocketing research in the field of nanoscience and nanotechnology. This new stream of science has proved itself to be worthy enough to be a part of multidisciplinary field of technology, which, in near future will grasp each and every corner of our life. Throughout the last decade, these nano particles have found applications in several sectors. Food and dairy processing industries are going through major shift in their technological approaches and nano science have attracted their attention too. In the area of food and dairy, the major utilities have been for food safety and bio security, packaging and nano-delivery systems (Chen *et al.,* 2006). Many products of nanoscience are already commercially, and they have received tremendous positive response from the users.

Confining solely to food and dairy sector, the additives fabricated in nano scale have effectively been responsible for improving the flavour and texture of the base food material and helped in enhancing their functionality. Implication of nano science in food packaging has resulted in the development of nano sensor based food packaging material having antimicrobial activators. Edible nano wrapper will help in enveloping foods thereby preventing gas and moisture exchange, which will help in extending shelf life by preventing early food spoilage (Miller, 2008; Richardson and Piehowski, 2008).

Nano particles can be prepared by top-down or bottom-up approach. The top down approach suggests the physical machining of the materials by milling, grinding, etching or lithography. In contrast to it, bottom-up approach indicates self-organization or self-assembly, that is, building up larger structures molecule by molecule or even atom by atom (Sozer and Kokini, 2008).

Nano particles have much more surface area; hence they show higher biological activity as compared to the macro particles of same composition. Thus, nano particles can effectively act as bioactive compounds in functional foods. Nano food applications can be classified into three broad categories namely- food additives, delivery systems and food packaging (Figure 10.1). This chapter gives a thorough overview of the areas of human interest influenced by nano science and its application in maintaining the quality of dairy and other food products.

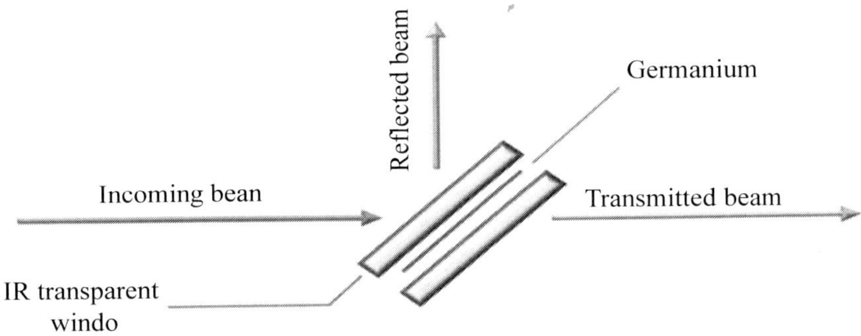

Fig. 10.1: Nano science and technology applications in dairy and food sector

Food Additives Applications

Nowadays, focus is given on fortifying food and dairy products with nano encapsulated nutrients. This kind of fortification is preferred over traditional ones because of improved colour, flavour, texture and even enhanced functional properties, apart from cutting down fat and sugar content. The particle size chosen is approximately 100 nm or less, which puts at ease the absorption of nutrients from the walls of stomach and intestine. The health food market and the sports supplements are the main target for this innovation.

Nanoceuticals

Nutraceuticals are the compounds which provide specialized health benefits beyond just basic nutrition required for growth and maintenance. Nano materials serve as bioactive compounds in functional foods (Chau *et al.,* 2007). Bringing down the size of particles to nanometer range aids in maintaining stability during processing, enhanced bioavailability, efficient delivery, better absorption, increased solubility and hence improved biological activity (Chen *et al.,* 2006). Nanoceuticals are of tremendous interest to the food and dairy processing sector ultimately benefitting the consumers. Carotenoids, omega-3 fatty acids, vitamins, minerals, lycopene and some probiotic species are few examples of the nanoparticles used in commercial productions of food/ dairy supplements. Nano sized supplements like pectin, inulin, polysaccharides (having surface active properties) used in functional butter (Ivanon and Rashevskaya, 2011) resulted in reduction of their structural elements to the range of 1-100 nm and modification of their architecture, structure and morphology.

Nanoencapsulation

Nano encapsulation is basically a type of encapsulation where, the functional ingredient is embedded into wall materials or vesicles of nanometer size. It offers several benefits like protection from damage or degradation during processing, controlled release and site-specific delivery, carrier or lipophilic nutrients, compatibility with other food ingredients and aiding in better absorption and enhanced bioavailability (Chen *et al.,* 2006), all of which leads to reduced usage of the main ingredient (Huang *et al.,* 2011). Thus, it can be claimed that the encapsulation by nanotechnology can improve the functionality and increase stability of the active ingredients manifold.

Delivery Systems Applications

The main role of this system is to carry the sensitive bioactive compound, protect them from getting degraded while being exposed to unfavourable conditions during food processing or in the gut and controlled the target specific release of active nutrients (Weiss *et al.,* 2006).

Association Colloids

Colloids are defined as stable systems where one kind of particles is in dispersed phase and the other one is in dispersed medium. Association colloids are nothing but colloidal systems having particle smaller particle size in the range of 5-100 nm. Few examples are surfactant micelles, reverse micelles, vesicles, bi-layers and liquid crystals which help in encapsulation and delivery of non polar, polar and even amphiphilic functional nutrients (Flanagan and Singh, 2006).

Biopolymeric Nano Particles

The biopolymeric nano materials forma a class of nano delivery systems. Food grade biopolymers like polysaccharides and proteins can undergo phase separation in mixed biopolymer systems or aggregation or self-association to produce nanoparticles (Gupta and Gupta, 2005). The combination of albumin and polyacrylamide and polymethylacrylate was first used to develop biopolymeric nanoparticles. Poly Lactic Acid has been used for encapsulation of several drugs and even iron or vitamin supplements. However, its performance enhances while being associated with polyethylene glycol and efficiently helps in triggering specific response (Riley *et al.,* 1999).

Nanoemulsion

Nano emulsions are different from conventional emulsions in the way that the diameter of the particles is in the range of 100-500 nm fabricated by using microfluidizers or high-pressure valve homogenizers. The bioactive compounds can be embedded within such droplets, in the continuous phase or even in the interfacial region. The nano structures are responsible for giving them unique textural and rheological properties by virtue of which, they seem transparent and pleasant to touch (Sonneville-Aubrun, 2004); which widens their utilities in food and cosmetic industries. The nano sized shell around the droplets can be engineered to develop them into smart delivery systems. Food ingredients like proteins, phospholipids and polysaccharides and processing operations like mixing and homogenization, which were already in use for making emulsions, are utilized for interfacial engineering technology (Weiss *et al.,* 2006). They provide several benefits like maintaining the same creaminess but with less usage of fat, thereby providing a healthier option for the aware consumers. The emulsions can be claimed to be more stable as the reduced size of droplets prevent the breaking of emulsion. Thus, use of certain stabilizers can be cut down. Low fat ice cream, spreads and mayonnaise having nano structure are already available in the market. Unilever and Nestle, the two giants of food industries have commercialized the nano-emulsion based ice creams having low fat content.

Nanotubes

Nano tubes are prepared from globular proteins of milk under suitable conditions by the bottom –up approach of self assembly. An appropriate example for this is the partially hydrolysed α-lactalbumin which is used for making nano tubes at a neutral pH by self-aggregation of the partially hydrolysed molecules in the presence of cations. The unique features offered by α-lactalbumin make it an excellent encapsulating agent and the nano tubes formed show a cavity diameter of 8 nm which helps in binding of vitamins, minerals and other food components (Srinivas *et al.,* 2010) and also masking of undesirable aroma or flavour. Being a milk protein, α-lactalbumin derived nano tubes can be easily applied.

Nanocapsules

Casein micelles in the milk have been designed by nature to act as a vehicle for proteins, calcium phosphate and other nutrients to the neonate. Their unique properties render them stable in adverse processing conditions and induce better absorption and digestibility (Gouin, 2004). A welcoming approach is the fortification of food and dairy products having low fat or non fat base with hydrophobic nutraceuticals which will not affect the sensory properties of the products. This could be achieved by their nano encapsulation before being incorporated into the food matrix.

Nano Precipitation Technique

When an internal organic phase containing the dissolved polymer and organic solvent is emulsified with external aqueous phase, which method is called nano precipitation technique. In this case, the polymer is precipitated from the organic medium and the organic solvent diffuses into the aqueous phase which promotes nanospheres and nanocapsules formation. The biodegradable polymers commonly used are poly (lactide) (PLA), polycaprolactone (PCL), poly (lactide-coglicolide) (PLGA), poly (alkylcyanoacrylate) (PACA) and Eudragit®. Curcumin, β-carotene and astaxanthin are few examples of bioactive compounds nano encapsulated using this technique. However, it must be kept in mind that the organic phase must be of food grade when used for food or dairy industry.

Food Packaging Applications

This is one the earliest and most widely used application of nano science in food and dairy industry. Till date, almost 500 nano packaging materials have already been approved for commercial use. It is expected that by the upcoming decade, about 25% of the packaging materials in the world will be substituted by nano structured ones. The main motto of such advanced packaging materials is to enhance the shelf life of the product by preventing mainly the exchange of oxygen and moisture (Sorrentino *et al.,* 2007).

Modified Atmospheric Packaging (MAP) involves the use of oxygen scavengers in food packages. Better the control of packaging materials on its moisture exchange properties and internal gas composition, higher the quality of that packaging material and the shelf life of the product can be increased by several weeks. Oxygen scavenging films can be made by adding titania nanorod particles (fabricated by titanium dioxide) to different polymers or by adding sharply defined layers (having nanometer thickness) to the ordinary paper or plastic packaging material. Clay nanoparticles can also be used for this purpose which adds reinforcing compounds to improve thermal and mechanical properties of the film.

Another application of nano science in packaging materials is that materials can be fabricated such that they release flavours, enzymes, antioxidants, antimicrobials and nutraceuticals. Natural antimicrobial agents can be impregnated to nano structured matrix, which will help in controlling the growth of spoilage causing and pathogenic organisms and extending food shelf-life. Silver has established antimicrobial properties and nano silver particles are already available in the market. However, there is room for the development and use of nano gold, nano copper oxide, nano magnesium oxide, nano chitosan, carbon nano tubes etc. in packaging materials in recent future.

Biodegradable Packaging

The alarming situation of the tremendous pollution globally has marked the way for increased inclination towards biodegradable packaging materials. They get degraded by metabolism of natural organisms and that too without the generation of any environmental hazard. They are produced by polymers directly extracted from biomass like protein, polysaccharides, peptides and polynucleotides. However, they have weak mechanical and barrier properties due to their hydrophilic nature. The use of nanotechnology can be used, whereby it can reduce the cost apart from the betterment of their physical properties (Lagaron *et al.,* 2005 and Sinha Ray and Bousmina, 2005). The major agents used for this are starch and derivatives, polyhydroxyl butyrate, poly lactide and aliphatic polyesters as polycaprolactone. Polylactide and starch based polymers have a combination of several properties which include low moisture barrier, low thermal stability, high mechanical strength. It has been observed that the use of clay (Avella *et al.,* 2005) in this case can help in reducing oxygen permeability as well as improving yield strength and tensile modulus.

Nano Coatings

Waxy coatings have been in use since many years to prevent moisture loss in case of fruits and vegetables (Park, 1999). However, it is a recent approach to use nanotechnology for development of nano scale edible coatings (5nm width). Apart from being a barrier to moisture loss, they also serve as a supplier of colour, flavour, antioxidant and antimicrobial compounds (Qureshi *et al.,* 2012). Several food products have been served with this technology like fruits, vegetables, meats, candies, chocolates and cheeses (Rhim, 2004).

Nano Laminates

Nano laminate is a special type of laminate film based on nanotechnology. It involves lamination using two or more layers of nanoscale width, which are strongly bonded to each other either by physical or by chemical means. Food and dairy sectors are exploring this novel technology. Weiss *et al.* (2006) suggested that nano lamination has more advantages as compared to conventional ones because of their unique property. Lipids, proteins, polysaccharides and micelles are the major substances used in this application by the simple method of washing and dipping. They have been successful in incorporating flavours, enzymes, antioxidants and antimicrobials, which have undoubtedly, lead to the extension of the products' shelf life.

Nano Fibres

Their diameters lie in the range of 10-1000 nm and they work as an excellent base for structural matrix of artificial foods as well as for bacterial cultures. Nano fibres can be produced by electrospin technology which employs applying to the solution a strong electric field specifically to a spinneret with a small capillary orifice (Figure 10.2). Apart from being used as a platform for structural matrix and nano structured scaffolding for cultures of different species of bacteria, they have several other applications. One of the most important of them being the building element of packaging material for green composite food.

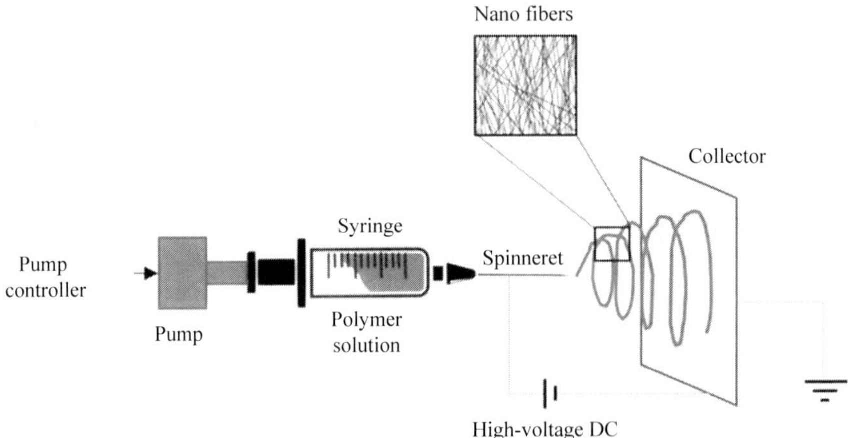

Fig. 10.2: Electrospinning process technology

Nano Sensors

It is a device comprising an electronic data processing part and a sensor. Its main work is to convert the signal of presence of light, gas or any organic substance into an electronic signal. These nano sensors can be used for assessing the quality of the food and dairy products and checking with the consumer acceptance. They function either by being incorporated directly into the food or its packaging material or even in the food processing equipments. In a way, the anno sensors may form important component of intelligent packaging systems. DNA-based biochips are a recent development in this sector. Electronic nose and electronic tongue are among few examples of such sensors. They can successfully detect the qualitative and quantitative presence of pathogens, toxins, allergens. They give results by changing their strip colour being highly sensitive to the gases evolved due to spoilage. However, few factors need to be kept in mind while commercializing their use. The most important among them being the cost and safety of materials to be used. The development of electronic barcodes as sensors is still at its infancy. More research is going on in this sector. Radio Frequency Identification Display is a next generation packaging display that consists of a microprocessor and an antenna that is capable of transmitting data to a wireless receiver. It is technologically more advanced that electronic tongue and bar codes. Smart antimicrobial packaging helps in absorbing oxygen thereby keeping food fresh for a long time (Clark, 2006). Ravichandran (2010), used nanotechnology for developing a bioswitch to operate 'release on command' preservative packaging.

Concerns Regarding Nano Science

The primary concern about nano particles is that, the macro compounds, which were generally recognized a safe (GRAS) may not be safe when used in nano sizes of the particles of same composition. Because of the increased surface area of the nano particles, studies should be conducted based upon their possible ill effects on health. These particles have more mobility, are more reactive, hence assumed to be toxic. Their properties, mainly, mass, particle size, surface properties and chemical composition influence human health. Studies like toxicology analysis, overall sustainability, recyclability and biological fate should be performed. The potential risks are assessed by the factors like the extension of penetration into human body, translocation and accumulation. Thus, regulatory systems capable of managing all kinds of risks involving nano particles should be established urgently.

Conclusion

Thus, in short, nano science has immense potentials and it shows promising applications in food production and processing industry. It also finds use during transportation, storage and concerning safety of food and dairy products. The dairy industry takes the benefit of using it as delivery vehicle for bioactive compounds, resulting in better absorption and enhanced bioavailability and also for the development of new and unique taste, sensory appeal, consistency and body texture and innovations in product packaging. This field is still at its infancy and enormous number of researches is going on to know deeper about this field of science. The world is still in dark about the health and environmental hazards (if any) of the nano particles. The field of nano science has been successful in the betterment of dairy quality throughout the world. Henceforth, the demand for both convenience and health can be met by the efficient use of nanotechnology in daily life. However, each and every factor including, consumer preference, government regulations, country's economy and environmental safety has to be considered which will ultimately decide the success of this advanced technology.

References

Avella, M., De Vlieger, J. J., Errico, M. E., Fischer, S., Vacca, P. & Volpe, M. G. (2005). Biodegradable starch/clay nanocomposite films for food packaging applications. *Food Chemistry*, 93(3): 467- 474.

Chau, C. F., Wu, S.H. & Yen, G.C. (2007). The development of regulation for food nanotechnology. *Trends in Biotechnology*, 27: 82-88.

Chavada, P. J. (2016). Novel application of nanotechnology in dairy and food industry: Nano inside. *International Journal of Agriculture Sciences*, 8(54): 2920-2922.

Chen, H., Weiss, J. & Shahidi, F. (2006). Nanotechnology in neutraceuticals and functional food technology. *Food Techology*, 60: 30-36.

Clark, J. P. (2006). Nanotechnology a processing topic this year. *Food Technology*, 60:135-140.

Flanagan, J., & Singh H. (2006). Microemulsions: a potential delivery system for bioactives in foods. *Critical Reviews in Food Science and Nutrition*, 46: 221-237.

Gouin, S. (2004). Micro-encapsulation: Industrial appraisal of existing technologies and trends. *Trends in Food Science and Technology*, 15: 330-347.

Gupta A.K. & Gupta, M. (2005). Synthesis and surface engineering of iron oxide nanoparticles for biomedical applications. *Biomaterials*, 26(18): 3995-4021.

Huang, Y., Chen, S., Bing, X., Gao, C., Wang, T. & Yuan, B. (2011). Nano silver migrated into food-simulating solutions from commercially available food fresh containers. *Packaging Technology and Science*, 24(5): 291-297.

Ivanov, S. V. & Rashevskaya, T. A. (2011). The nanostructure's management is the basis for a functional fatty food's production. *Proceedia Food Science*, 1: 24- 31.

Lagaron, J. M., Cabedo, L., Cava, D., Feijoo, J. L., Gavara, R., & Gimenez, E. (2005). Improving packaged food quality and safety. Part 2: nanocomposites. *Food Additives and Contaminants*, 22(10), 994-998.

Miller, G. (2008). Nanotechnology- the new threat to food. http://www.globalresearch.ca/index.php?context=va& aid=10755 (last access on 21/8/2020)

Nickols-Richardson, N. S. M. & Piehowski, K.E. (2008). Nanotechnology in nutritional sciences. *Minerva Biotechnologica*, 20: 117-126.

Park, H. J. (1999). Development of advanced edible coatings for fruits. *Trends in Food Science and Technology*, 10: 254-260.

Qureshi, M. A., Karthikeyan, S., Karthikeyan, P., Ahmed, P. A., Uprit, S. & Mishra, U. K. (2012). Application of nanotechnology in food and dairy processing: An overview. *Pakistan Journal of Food Science*, 22: 23-31.

Ravichandran, R. (2010). Nanoparticles in drug delivery: potential green nano biomedicine applications. *International Journal of Green Nanotechnology Biomedicine*, 1: 108-130.

Ravichandran, R. & Sasi, K. P. (2006). Nanoscience and nanotechnology: perspectives and overview. *First Indian at the South Pole 3 PS Sehra Madame Marie Curie–Radioactivity and 10 Atomic Energy*, 44(2): 43-49

Rhim, J. W. (2004). Increase in water vapor barrier property of biopolymerbased edible films and coatings by compositing with lipid materials. *Food Science and Biotechnology*, 13: 528-535.

Riley, T., T., Govender, S., Stolnik, C.D., Xiong, M.C., Garnett, L., Illum & Davis, S. S. (1999). Colloidal stability and drug incorporation aspects of micellar like PLA-PEG nanoparticles. *Colloids and Surfaces. B. Biointerfaces*, 16: 147-159.

Sinha Ray, S. & Bousmina, M. (2005). Biodegradable polymers and their layered silicate nanocomposites: in greening the 21st century materials world. *Progress in Materials Science*, 50(8): 962-1079.

Sonneville-Aubrun, O., Simonnet, J. T. & L'Alloret, F. (2004). Nanoemulsions: a new vehicle for skincare products. *Advances in Colloid and Interface Science*, 108: 145-149

Sorrentino, A., Gorrasi, G. & Vittoria, V. (2007). Potential perspectives of bionanocomposites for food packaging applications. *Trends in Food Science and Technology*, 18(2): 84-95.

Sozer, N. & Kokini, J. L. (2008). Nanotechnology and its applications in the food sector. *Trends in Biotechnology*, 27: 82-88.

Srinivas, P.R., Philbert, M., Vu, T.Q., Huang, Q., Kokini, J. L. & Saos, E. (2010). Nanotechnology research applications in nutritional sciences. *The Journal of Nutrition*, 140:119-124.

Weiss, J., Paul, T. Julian, D. & McClements, D. J. (2006). Functional materials in Food nanotechnology. *Journal of Food science*, 71: 107-116.

11

Nutrigenomics and Milk: A Perspective

Shikha Pandhi, Veena Paul and Arvind

Department of Dairy Science and Food Technology, Institute of Agricultural Sciences, Banaras Hindu University, Varanasi, India

Abstract

The fascinating area of nutrigenomics defines the interaction between food-nutrients, their metabolites, and our genome. In the dairy industry, the application of nutrigenomics is an emerging area of research. The nutrients can interrelate by genes and modifies molecular mechanisms affecting physical properties. This has directed to an emerging interest among scientists in discovering nutrient-gene interaction at the molecular level that affect the dairy industry's nutrigenomics. Dietary supplements also play a crucial part in nutrigenomics as the nutrients influence the gene expression. Researchers are exploring the application of nutrigenomics in the dairy industry, mainly for the milk-fat synthesis and milk-protein synthesis. This chapter aims to provide an overview of nutrigenomics and its application in the dairy industry. This chapter emphasizes nutrient-gene interaction by employing nutrigenomics research tools like transcriptomics, metabolomics, and proteomics. This chapter also focuses on the application of nutrigenomics in milk, ruminants, and animal nutrition.

Introduction

The exploration of facts about healthy and nutritious food has increased over the years. The advent of advance scientific tools has elucidated facts regarding the role of diet or nutrients in regulating gene expression (Sales *et al.,* 2014). Various studies based on molecular interactions in food has revealed that many dietary components such as proteins, carbohydrates, fats, minerals, vitamins and phyto-constituents has the tendency to regulate gene expression. The science that studies the interaction of dietary components with the genes to modify the phenotype and nutrient metabolism is known as "Nutrigenomics" (Zdunczyk and Pareek, 2009). The word "nutrigenomics" is an amalgamation of two words “nutri” (stands for nutrient) and “genomics.” It studies the “genome-wide influence of nutrients” and how they alter the sense of equilibrium among health and illness through modification of gene expression or an individual’s genomic makeup (Neeha and Kinth, 2013). The science of nutrigenomics uses high-throughput ‘omics’ technologies like metabolomics, proteomics, and transcriptomics to study nutrition’s influence on health and well-being (Zdunczyk and Pareek, 2009). Nutrigenomics has come up as an important area in nutritional research over the years. It plays a critical part in revealing the role of various nutrients and food constituents in preventing obesity, cardiovascular diseases, and cancer prevention. From a nutrigenomic viewpoint, dietary nutrients serve as signals which are identified by the cells sensing system affecting the gene expression and, consequently, metabolite generation (Muller and Kersten, 2003). From the research point of view, tools like transcriptomics, proteomics, and metabolomics play a crucial role in studying the influence of dietary nutrients on gene (Zdunczyk and Pareek, 2009).

In general, a nutrigenomic study delivers a clear snapshot of how genes are turned on or off at any point of time and describe how gene/nutrient interacts with each other to yield a specific response. It is assumed that strengthening the understanding of this field will provide a better representation of how nutritients affects homeostasis and eventually aids in preventing chronic diseases (Neeha and Kinth, 2013). Nutrigenomics in conjugation with milk is a relatively new area of research. Given the prospects mentioned above of this science in the nutritional study, the present book chapter tends to present a perspective on the application of nutrigenomics in milk and dairy sector, which is less explored.

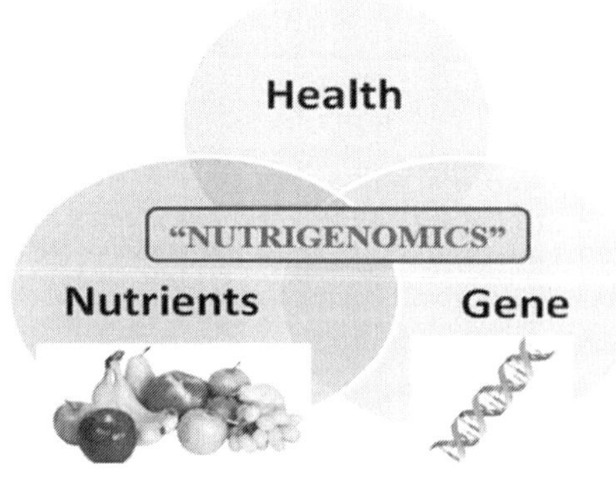

Fig. 11.1: Nutrigenomics approach

Nutrient-Gene Interaction

Nutrigenomics denotes the nutrient-gene interaction and their influence on gene expression. The gene expression is influenced by nutrients at different levels of transcription, translation, and post-translation. In the nutrient-gene interaction, the nutrition intake in diet changes the gene expression without altering the DNA sequence (Dauncey, 2012). The nutrient-gene interaction deals with how nutrition affects the gene function and vice versa. The interaction among the body and nutrition is a complex process as it encompasses molecular mechanisms for regulating genes. Nutrients that are consumed by organisms worked as nascent signals that regulate the synthesis pathway and acts as storage during starvation (Cahill and Rimm, 2015; Corthesy-Theulaz *et al.*, 2005; Torronen *et al.*, 2006). These nutrients, after consumption, are digested and bio-transform by several proteins in the body. This leads to polymorphisms in genes encoding these proteins altering proteins' functioning (Cahill and Rimm, 2015). Nutrients are the external factors that send metabolic signals to the nucleus linked to genes. The organism responds to genes encoding cell differentiation, cell growth, and energy metabolism via these metabolic signals. Thus, the nutrient-gene interaction is linked with organisms' dietary intake as a lack of a balanced diet alters the interaction leading to the risk of developing chronic diseases (Torronen *et al.*, 2006).

The expression of genetic information is controlled by nutrients present in food. The genomes are affected by several environmental factors (like physiological and psychological stress), which hinders genetic information (Dauncey, 2012; Torronen *et al.*, 2006). The dietary components have the potential to alter the genetic events, and thus affecting the health. Health is influence by the number of essential nutrients like carbohydrate, protein, vitamins, minerals, and bioactive components, which control the gene expression in response to nutritional changes (Corthesy-Theulaz *et al.*, 2005; Torronen *et al.*, 2006). These nutrients are responsible for modifying the cellular process linked with disease prevention that involves hormonal balance, apoptosis, cell signaling, and carcinogen metabolism. Genetics can influence the food preference of an individual. For instance, the TAS2R38 gene encodes bitter taste receptors present in the tongue (taste buds). Due to polymorphism, it causes an individual to experience a bitter taste differently. Brussels sprouts seem to be bitter to some individuals while some individuals cannot taste the bitterness. Some individuals can taste phenylthiocarbamide and 6-n-propylthiouracil (bitter compounds) that can influence the TAS2R38 gene (Khataan *et al.*, 2009; Mennella *et al.*, 2010; Torronen *et al.*, 2006).

In the nutrient-gene interaction, the nutrients acted directly as ligands for transcription factors and metabolized by the metabolic pathway for gene regulation. From the molecular perspective, nutrients are considered signaling molecules responsible for translating dietary signals to gene, protein, and metabolite expression via cellular sensing mechanisms (Afman and Muller, 2006; Torronen *et al.,* 2006). The sensor pathways involved in the interaction can also be influenced by structural changes of nutrients (like saturated and unsaturated fatty acids). The nutrient-gene interaction is of three types: (1) Direct interactions – In this type of interaction, the nutrients behave as transcription factors. (2) Epigenetic interactions – This type of interaction alters the DNA structure by altering the gene expression. (3) Genetic Variations – This type of interaction involves several genetic variations that can alter the gene expression (Siddique *et al.,* 2009).

The main link of nutrient-gene interaction is transcription, which influences the gene expression (Muller and Kersten, 2003; Ordovas, 2006; Torronen *et al.,* 2006). The transcription factor consists of a nuclear receptor that acts as a nutrient sensor by binding nutrients with metabolites. For instance, peroxisome proliferator-activated receptors (PPAR) bind fatty acids. These receptors, when get activated, enable the nutrients to influence specific genes. Nutrigenomics deals with the interaction of the genome and its nutritional conditions. This nutrient-gene interaction, thus, guides the balance between nutrient and gene required to maintain the optimal health of an individual (Torronen *et al.,* 2006).

Nutrigenomics Research Tools

The advancement of nutrigenomics has made use of novel research tools such as transcriptomics, proteomics, and metabolomics for food research and animal nutrition studies (Zdunczyk and Pareek, 2009). These tools provide nutritionists with genetic backgrounds to screen the transcriptome, proteome, and metabolome. The information gathered using these tools can be utilized to develop a dietary strategy that facilitates the targeted nutrition supply to the individuals (Neeha and Kinth, 2013). The transcriptome is a complete array of RNA molecules expressed by an organism. The science of transcriptomics deals with the study of gene expression at mRNA level (transcriptome). This approach can be utilized to analyse gene expression of a biological specimen under specified conditions and time frame with the application of cDNA or oligonucleotide microarray technique. Transcriptomics is the most extensively employed 'omics' tool for nutrigenomic studies. The regulation of gene transcription rate by dietary constituents' acts as a stimulating locates for regulating an individual's phenotype. Dietary constituents can also greatly influence the translation process of converting RNA to protein as well as post-translational procedures that can influence the activity of protein. Further, proteomics deals with the proteome's study and talks about three classes of biological importance, such as expression, structure and function of proteins (Kussmann *et al.,* 2006). It tries to illustrate all the proteins present within a biological specimen and their comparative abundance, distribution, post-translational alterations, functions, and collaborations with other biological constituents. The science of proteomics is theoretically very thought-provoking, and the presence or absence of protein is not nearly suggestive of a metabolic modification. The newest of these "omics" tools in nutrigenomic is metabolomics that deals with the study of metabolites, the metabolome. It attempts to quantify all the constituents (apart from protein, RNA and DNA) in a given sample. A metabolome reveals the entire array of metabolites present in a given biological sample. The metabolomics study scrutinizes the whole metabolic route, which eventually indicates the effect of different genes. It examines metabolic regulation and fluctuations in cells due to a particular change in environmental conditions. Metabolomics is also a non-targeted determination method under specific environmental conditions similar to proteomics and transcriptomics (Torronen *et al.,* 2006).

Application of Nutrigenomics in Milk

Nowadays, nutrigenomics has its potential use in the field of nutrition research. These are applied to study the effect of nutrients and diet in cell models, experimental animals, and humans. Recently, the application of nutrigenomics in dairy cattle is a exploring area of research. The dietary habits of dairy cows are responsible for the alteration in gene expression. In dairy cows, nutrigenomics controls the responses by multiple transcription factors. The level of amino acids and fatty acids in cow feed has excellent potential. They are responsible for altering gene expression leading to the synthesis of milk fat by inhibiting the SREBP1 gene (Bionaz *et al.,* 2015).

The application of nutrigenomics in dairy cows is mainly made to improve milk fat by synthesizing the milk fat by trans-10 cis-12 CLA (conjugated linoleic acid isomers). Nutrient-gene interaction leads to whole-organism metabolism (Osorio and Moisa, 2019).

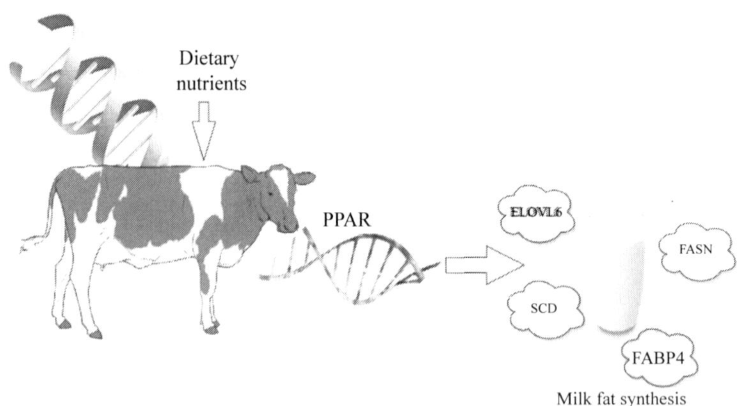

Fig. 11.2: Nutrigenomics in Dairy Cow

(ELOVL6: Fatty acid elongase 6; FASN: Fatty acid synthase; FABP4: Fatty acid binding protein 4; SCD: Stearoyl CoA desaturase; PPAR: peroxisome proliferator-activated receptors)

Application of Nutrigenomics in Ruminants

Dietary modification and improved nutritional strategies are the critical elements for enhancing the production and production quality in ruminants. Nutritional management is primarily crucial during the transition period and initial lactation phase when the animal is more prone to nutritional inequities. Exploring various nutrients that regulate the production and production quality in ruminants has been effectively studied using nutrigenomic studies. Improvement in milk fat is one such essential application. Multiple conjugated linoleic acid isomers have been shown to suppress the milk fat synthesis in the cow. This reduction in milk fat is mainly occurred during ruminal biohydrogenation under specified dietary conditions. During this diet-induced fat depression phase, there is no modification in the animal whole metabolism, but there is a decrease in the lipid synthesis capacity (Banupriya *et al.,* 2016).

Application of Nutrigenomics in Animal Nutrition

The conventional animal nutrition studies emphasize on nutrient deficiency management, nutrient associations and animal responses towards a particular dietary nutrient or feed. The emergence of nutrigenomic science and tools has helped to enhance the efficiency of farm animals' nutrition processes using updated technological interventions. Nutrigenomic studies can play an essential role in revealing the role of nutrients as dietary signals that are identified by the cells or tissues to modulate gene expression. These studies can be useful in identifying the markers responsible for a specific gene expression through the use of dietary nutrients with an overall aim to increase the production quality and animal performance (Asmare and Negewo, 2019).

Future Prospects

The balanced diet plays a significant role in maintaining health, as these are based on clinical, epidemiological, and experimental studies of different groups of individuals. In the past few years, a novel approach for studying human mechanism has been developed. The science of nutrigenomics has brought a new era to nutritional research by exploring the nutrient-gene interaction that modifies or determine the genetic factor. This interaction is based on the genetic make-up of an individual and the development of omics. Nutrigenomics aims to understand the physiology and disease via molecular pathways and their regulatory network in the body yielding health benefits by nutrient-gene interactions with new diagnostic tests related to diet-response. Thus, nutrigenomics has the potential to be a new biomarker for nutritional diseases. The genes responsible for disease progression can be employed as biomarkers for different diseases, and the genes and molecular pathways used as disease prevention targets. Knowing genes and their metabolic pathways and their pathogenesis role will give a novel approach to preventing disease. Nutrigenomics offers new opportunities in biochemistry, molecular biology, genetics, bioinformatics, and nutrition. Nutrigenomics offers an easier understanding of molecular approaches, and the effect of dietary intake on health will emphasize the need for training for students in clinical nutrition. Nutrigenomics also offers the creation of personalized diets based on the nutrition required to maintain individual health.

Moreover, advances have been made in understanding the diet-disease relation to prevent disease by dietary intervention. Moreover, research advancement in analytical and computational science will transform nutrition more systematically. The application of novel technologies in nutritional research, collaborative actions, and networks will be necessary.

Conclusion

Nutrigenomics is a novel approach in nutritional science that reveals how food interacts with the genes and how the organism reacts to these interactions through various tools such as transcriptomics, proteomics, and metabolomics. Although this nutrigenomics field is an extensive growing field still it is in its beginning phase especially in the milk and dairy domain. It has shown the ability to maintain animal well-being, optimize animal output and enhance the quality of milk. The supplementation of animal diets with different nutrients has shown to affect the milk composition. There is a growing need for a better understanding of how dietary nutrients affect the physiological processes and characteristics to acquire a desirable advantage for nutritional management. Further innovations require targeted study of specific genes to achieve desired output and performance in composition, production and production quality.

References

Afman, L. & Muller, M. (2006). Nutrigenomics: from molecular nutrition to prevention of disease. *Journal of the American Dietetic Association*, 106(4): 569–576.

Asmare, B., & Negewo, T. (2019). The Potential of nutrigenomics from viewpoint of animal nutrition: A mini review. *SVU-International Journal of Veterinary Sciences*, 2(1): 75-81.

Banupriya, S., Kathirvelan, C., & Joshua, P. P. (2016). Application of nutrigenomics for milk fat improvement in dairy cattle. *International Journal of Science, Environment and Technology*, 5(3): 1570 – 1573.

Bionaz, M., Osorio, J. & Loor, J. J. (2015). Triennial Lactation Symposium: Nutrigenomics in dairy cows: nutrients, transcription factors, and techniques. *Journal of Animal Science*, 93(12): 5531–5553.

Cahill, L. E. & Rimm, E. B. (2015). diet–gene interactions: haptoglobin genotype and nutrient status. In *Preventive Nutrition* (pp. 115–129). Springer.

Corthesy-Theulaz, I., den Dunnen, J. T., Ferre, P., Geurts, J. M. W., Muller, M., van Belzen, N. & van Ommen, B. (2005). Nutrigenomics: the impact of biomics technology on nutrition research. *Annals of Nutrition and Metabolism*, 49(6): 355–365.

Dauncey, M. J. (2012). Recent advances in nutrition, genes and brain health. *Proceedings of the Nutrition Society*, 71(4): 581–591.

Khataan, N. H., Stewart, L., Brenner, D. M., Cornelis, M. C. & El-Sohemy, A. (2009). TAS2R38 genotypes and phenylthiocarbamide bitter taste perception in a population of young adults. *Lifestyle Genomics*, 2(4–5): 251–256.

Kussmann, M., Raymond, F., & Affolter, M. (2006). OMICS-driven biomarker discovery in nutrition and health. *Journal of Biotechnology*, 124(4): 758-787.

Mennella, J. A., Pepino, M. Y., Duke, F. F. & Reed, D. R. (2010). Age modifies the genotype-phenotype relationship for the bitter receptor TAS2R38. *BMC Genetics*. 11(1): 60.

Müller, M. & Kersten, S. (2003). Nutrigenomics: goals and strategies. *Nature Reviews Genetics*, 4(4): 315–322.

Neeha, V. S. & Kinth, P. (2013). Nutrigenomics research: a review. *Journal of Food Science and Technology*, 50(3): 415-428.

Ordovas, J. M. (2006). Nutrigenetics, plasma lipids, and cardiovascular risk. *Journal of the American Dietetic Association*, 106(7): 1074–1081.

Osorio, J. S. & Moisa, S. J. (2019). Gene regulation in ruminants: A nutritional perspective. In *Gene Expression and Control*. IntechOpen, 1-27.

Sales, N. M. R., Pelegrini, P. B. & Goersch, M. C. (2014). Nutrigenomics: definitions and advances of this new science. *Journal of Nutrition and Metabolism*, 1-6.

Siddique, R. A., Tandon, M., Ambwani, T., Rai, S. N. & Atreja, S. K. (2009). Nutrigenomics: nutrient-gene interactions. *Food Reviews International*, 25(4): 326–345.

Torronen, R., Kolehmainen, M. & Poutanen, K. (2006). Nutrigenomics–new approaches for nutrition, food and health research. *Food and Health Research Centre*, 1–43.

Zdunczyk, Z., & Pareek, C. S. (2009). Application of nutrigenomics tools in animal feeding and nutritional research. *Journal of Animal and Feed Sciences*, 18(1): 3-16.

12

Metabolomics to Determine the Quality and Traceability of Milk

***Akshay Ramani*[1], *Ankitkumar J. Thesiya*[2], *Amit P. Patel*[2] and *Nikunj M. Vachhani*[2]**

[1]*Dairy Chemistry Division, ICAR-National Dairy Research Institute Karnal, Haryana, India*
[2]*College of Dairy Science, Kamdhenu University, Amreli, Gujarat, India*

Abstract

Metabolomics is a useful technique in dairy science. Metabolomics is concerned with identifying and quantifying the small molecules involved in metabolic reactions. Recently, it has been used to determine the nutritional content and authenticity of milk and milk products. During milk processing, transportation, and storage, metabolomics can aid in maintaining and enhancing product quality. Additionally, metabolite profiles obtained using metabolomics can detect chemical or biological contamination in dairy products. To identify and quantify the metabolites present in milk and milk products, various analytical techniques used such as NMR spectroscopy, LC-MS, GC-MS, and UPLC-QTOF mass spectrometry have been successfully used. This study focuses on current breakthroughs in metabolomics for milk and milk product quality and safety evaluations.

Keywords: Milk, Metabolomics, Spectroscopy, Quality

Introduction

Milk, commonly referred to as the "ideal food," is an essential source of nutrition for human consumption. Because of the growing human population and the rising demand for milk and milk products, there is more interest in and concern about the quality and safety of dairy products. Milk comprises chemical substances with various functions in the human body, such as carbohydrates, lipids, proteins, and trace elements (vitamins, minerals, etc.) (Guetouache *et al.*, 2014). Similar to milk proteins, bioactive peptides, fatty acids, nucleotides, and other nutrients have received significant study in dairy science. These so-called metabolites are the end products of cellular activity in organisms (dairy animals) and are directly related to phenotypes and changed biological condition and functions. Milk's quality can be affected by numerous factors, such as its chemical composition and metabolism, which can be influenced by genetics, diet, seasons, geographic origins, health of animals (healthy or sick), processing, storage, contamination, and adulteration. Milk's chemical composition and microbial responses can be altered by processing effects (such as thermal processing, fermentation, storage, etc.) (Suh, 2022). Metabolite profiles may be altered if products are contaminated or adulterated during production, transportation, or storage. Figure 12.1 depicts the factors that influence the quality of milk from the farm to the final products. Milk and milk product's chemical composition can indicate nutritional quality and safety, and some metabolites can be used to ensure quality assurance (e.g., authentication) and enhancement of product.

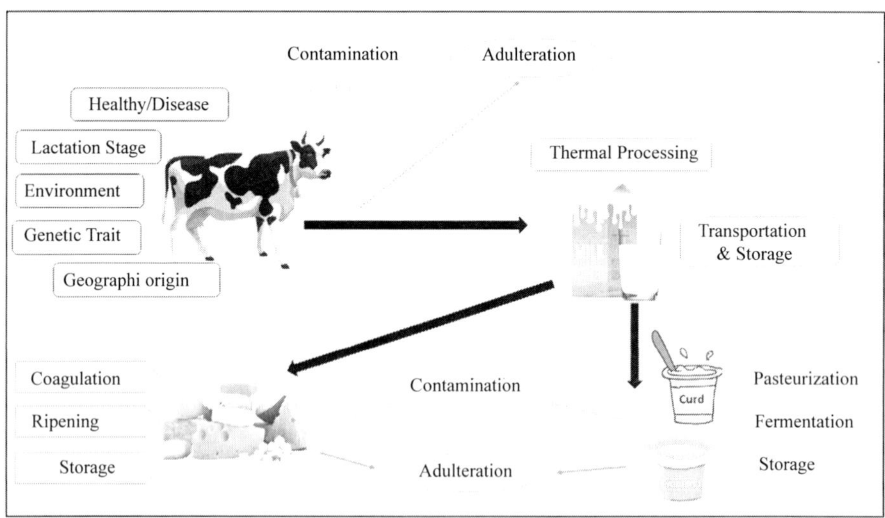

Fig. 12.1: Factors influencing the milk and milk products' quality

Metabolomics is the gold standard for identifying and quantifying the chemical composition of metabolites produced by diverse biological processes (Xiao *et al.*, 2012). Utilizing analytical tools such as mass spectrometry (MS) and nuclear magnetic resonance (NMR) spectroscopy, instrumental analyses are frequently necessary for the metabolomics method. Metabolomics is widely used in clinical and pharmaceutical science because it can cover a wide range of metabolites and has a high throughput. It is also being used more and more in other fields, such as food, nutrition, and plant science. The increasing application of metabolomics in the food and nutrition domains was instrumental in coining the name "Foodomics." In the past two years, research into the metabolomics of dairy products has exploded. This demonstrates that metabolomics has become a significant research tool for milk and milk products.

Metabolomics

The study of metabolomics involves a detailed analysis, both qualitatively and quantitatively, of all the small molecules present in an organism. Metabolomics tools are being used more and more to make unbiased global profiles of metabolites in samples (i.e., "untargeted analysis") or to measure a small panel of metabolites with high sensitivity (targeted analysis). By examining the metabolome of various bodily fluids from a dairy cow, numerous possible biomarkers of milk production and quality have been identified. One benefit of profiling metabolites is that it helps researchers figure out how the body's metabolism affects overall health (Sun *et al.*, 2015). This is accomplished by monitoring the process by which substances found in the blood, faeces, and diet are formed and broken down. It can also assess how well feed is utilised, how an animal's metabolism responds to the environment, and production efficiency and carcass quality attributes. Water-soluble molecules in beef, such as free amino acids, nucleotides, and sugars, have a heritability of less than 0.30 and vary with animal age, according to research (Carrillo *et al.*, 2016). However, these water-soluble chemicals were connected to a lower carcass weight and a lower beef marbling standard at the genetic level.

Thus, metabolomics could assist breeders identify animals with high-quality meat. In a separate investigation, metabolic profiling of muscle by GC-MS and LC-MS revealed with 100% accuracy which calves were given grass and which were fed grain (Sakuma *et al.*, 2017). These findings show that metabolic fingerprints may be a reliable method for determining what animals consume and the quality of their meat, thus they might be used to choose animals with desirable characteristics.

The developing breeding technology of metabolomic selection is based on nuclear magnetic resonance (NMR) or LC-MS metabolomics (Lippa *et al.*, 2022). Biological samples' NMR spectra can be studied for chemical shifts, peak intensities, and coupling patterns to identify and quantify specific metabolites and develop NMR fingerprints of the sample. Studies of the metabolites in the muscle and fat from cattle, pigs, and poultry have revealed tissue and species-specific variations in metabolites, with distinct chemicals found in each species (Ueda *et al.*, 2019). The GC-MS could also differentiate various breeds of cattle (Chakraborty *et al.*, 2022). Comparing the NMR spectra of various animals, such as those of low-performing and high-performing animals, may therefore aid in the identification of NMR fingerprints in high-performing animals. These NMR fingerprints can subsequently be utilized for the genetic selection and breeding of animals. High-growth animals exhibited a particular metabolic profile with a greater concentration of certain metabolites impacting protein and fatty acid metabolism, which can be utilized for the selection of animals for growth (Chakraborty *et al.*, 2022).

High-resolution MS (HRMS) can give a better picture of the metabolite landscape than NMR because it can find metabolites at concentrations from nano-molar to pico-molar (Goldansaz *et al.*, 2017; Hofmann, 2017). Depending on how polar and lipophilic the target metabolites are, the MS is often used with capillary, liquid, or gas chromatography to separate them. The separated molecules are ionised by ESI, electron ionisation (EI), chemical ionisation (CI), or atmospheric pressure chemical ionisation (APCI), and then the m: z ratio is checked in a mass spectrometer based on TOF, Fourier transformation ion cyclotron resonance (FT-ICR), or orbitrap. This gives structural data that can be used to identify the metabolites. Metabolites can be identified by comparing their MS spectra to those in databases like METLIN, the Human Metabolome Database (HMDB), and MassBank. Then, various statistical and bioinformatics tools can be employed to identify the metabolic pathways that lead to the formation of these essential metabolites. Metabolic pathways can be examined and comprehended using tools such as MetaboAnalyst and the Kyoto Encyclopaedia of Genes and Genomes (KEGG). Finding metabolic markers associated with performance for genetic selection may be aided by the correlation analysis between animal performance indicators and metabolic profiles. In GWAS, metabolomics has also been applied to phenotyping and animal breeding based on metabolite profiles (Fontanesi, 2016).

The accuracy of genetic selection and animal breeding can be increased by combining metabolomics technologies with molecular breeding tools like WGS and high-density SNP chips (Wang & Kadarmideen, 2020). Genomic prediction can estimate breeding values based on phenotype and pedigree, but genomic data alone cannot indicate an animal's genetic potential. Adding whole-metabolomic data may increase the genetic gain by making selection more precise. Metabolites are the final physiological response of a cell, and they link the genotype to the phenotype (Chakraborty *et al.*, 2022). In GWAS-based research, SNP chips and LC-MS metabolomics were used to figure out how the genetic differences in pigs affect how well they use feed. Also, it has been found that combining high-density SNP data with information about metabolites that has predictive value can help improve the accuracy of genetic selection in cattle. With the help of new types of bio-samples like semen, amniotic fluid, saliva, and urine, metabolomics can find small changes in phenotype, innate phenotype tendencies, and nutritional responses in livestock research, breeding, and evaluation without harming the animals.

According to Wu (2021), the small metabolite profiling of pig faeces by LC-MS metabolomics revealed a correlation between the animals' feed efficiency and their ability to respond to new feed additives. This information can be used to help select animals that have high feeding efficiency. Given that the metabolites found in the faeces are reflections of the intestinal microbiota, cellular metabolism, and the digestion and absorption of nutrients in the gut, they may be a good indicator of the efficiency with which the animal converts its feed. In beef cattle, it has also been demonstrated that stress alters the faecal metabolome. Since "metabolic fingerprints" are known to exist in animals with high feed conversion efficiency or stress tolerance, metabolic profiling of faecal matter may be used to identify those animals (Yoon *et al.*, 2021). Then, this animal can be chosen for breeding. The impact of genetic selection on indirect genetic effects (IGE) in breeding programmes has also been investigated using metabolomics (Dervishi *et al.*, 2021). Future metabolomics studies may combine a variety of analytical methods (such as ICP-MS, MSI, and fluxomics) with multi-omics experiments to provide more precise data. More sensitive platforms, such ESI-MS, may be used.

Metabolomics is the study of small molecules found in animals, plants, and microorganisms termed metabolites. By comparing metabolome profiles (metabolic phenotypes or "metabotypes"), it is possible to identify patterns of differences between different groups, such as control vs treatment, healthy vs sick-diseased. Significant breakthroughs have been made in animal welfare, reproduction, and development as a result of metabolomics. It has also assisted in identifying biomarkers for mutating illnesses and productivity features in dairy and meat cattle. All of these measures are taken to increase the accuracy of predictive approaches in animal health. In addition, numerous biofluids, including as plasma, milk, urine, and serum, have been investigated for metabolomics studies. This has helped lessen animal welfare concerns. Two primary methods are utilised today in metabolomics, specifically, mass spectrometry (MS) and nuclear magnetic resonance (NMR) spectrometry. Mass spectrometry, however, is typically paired in conjunction with a method of separation, such gas chromatography (GC), Chromatography in a liquid medium (LC) or capillary electrophoresis (CE). Nuclear magnetic resonance (NMR) is now a more advanced method than mass spectrometry. MS allows for the rapid assessment of large samples at a low cost per sample. The time required to obtain an NMR spectrum is 5-8 minutes, whereas the time required to obtain an IR spectrum is substantially less (between 5 and 30 minutes). Because to the high sensitivity of mass spectrometry (MS), it can detect a larger range of coverage. More innovative technologies are being developed to take use of its potential benefits in terms of metabolites per minute than nuclear magnetic resonance (NMR). A number of advances in the field of metabolomics have occurred in recent years. Technological advancements and trends that are faster and more efficient comprehensive processing with lower samples at an acceptable cost-per-sample. New information Initiatives to exchange information and standardised data reporting will make it simpler to adopt completely automated data analysis tools based on open source software to use the massive amounts of information obtained from omics studies to new biological understanding.

Integrating omics and phenotypic data in metabolomics is difficult. Examining new samples, such as saliva, urine, amniotic fluid, and sperm, and adding more animal breeds might improve metabolome research.

Methods for Milk and Dairy Product Metabolomics Analysis

A viable strategy for determining the milk's overall quality and authenticity is to characterise its metabolome. Characterizing the milk metabolome can help determine its quality and authenticity. The metabolomic fingerprint of milk and dairy products can be obtained using GC-MS, NMR, HRMAS NMR, LC-MS, and LC-MS/MS (Rocchetti & O'Callaghan, 2021). These methodologies use analytical instruments with differing sensitivity and metabolite coverage. In milk metabolomics research, NMR is the most prevalent analytical platform (Pan *et al.*, 2018). NMR is frequently used because of its dependability and usefulness in absolute quantitation, however it is highly insensitive and only capable of measuring compounds at concentrations between micromolar and millimolar (Sen *et al.*, 2021). However, MS-based technologies (such LC-MS and LC-MS/MS) can recognise metabolites at nanomolar to picomolar concentrations, enabling the detection of a significantly higher number of metabolites. Additionally, GC-MS is more reliable and reproducible than LC-MS but is less sensitive. As a result, GC-MS offers greater accuracy and repeatability than either NMR or LC-MS in the identification and quantification of milk metabolites. Comprehensive metabolomics profiles are produced using LC-MS and GC-MS, especially for tiny metabolites (1-2 kDa) in complicated matrices (Sen *et al.*, 2021). It is obvious that each methodology has benefits and drawbacks, and frequently the methods work best together. To get the highest amount of metabolomic coverage, a combination method that uses more than one instrumental approach is most frequently recommended.

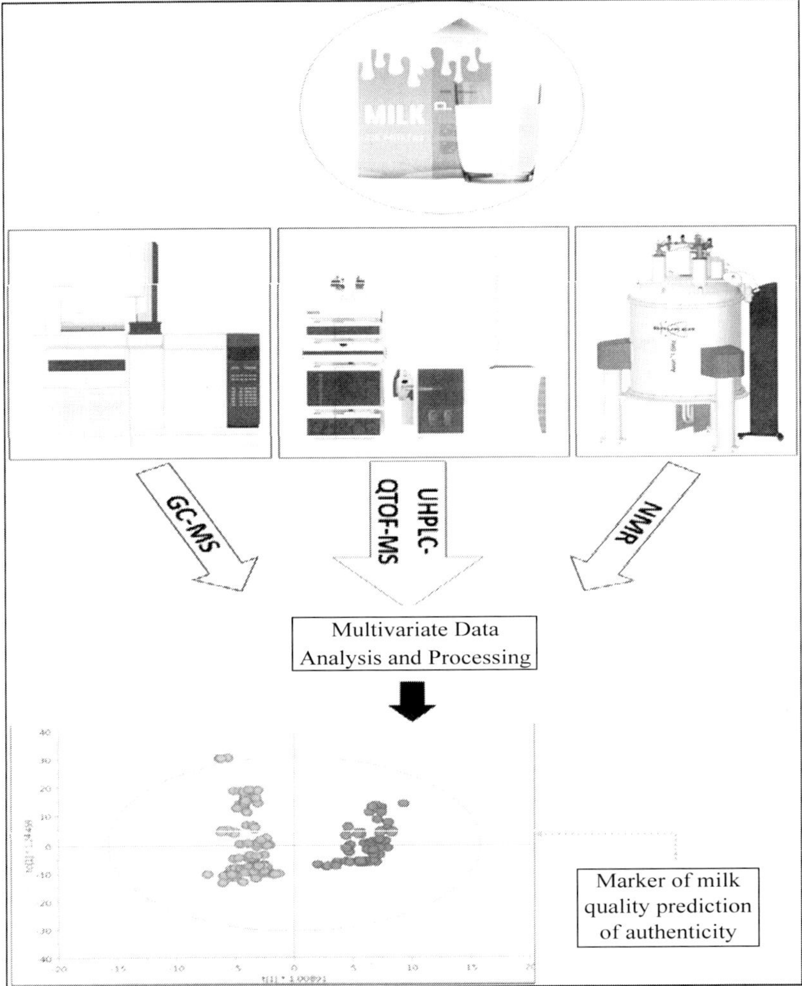

Fig. 12.2 Presents a summary of the most significant platforms for milk metabolomics.

Milk Metabolites for Herd Health Prediction

Use of Milk Metabolites in Herd Health Prediction

In recent years, there has been a greater emphasis on the development of technologies to anticipate animals' health and welfare condition rapidly and non-invasively, which can have significant implications for milk supply and quality. Several approaches have been proposed in the past, including rapid mid-infrared spectrometry analysis of milk samples for the prediction of energy balance and rapid detection of somatic cell counts (SCC) in milk, which has been widely used for many years as a predictor of the presence of mastitis in the cow's udder. Sundekilde (2013) found a substantial relationship between milk SCC and its metabolite profile, with increasing SCC raising levels of lactate, butyrate, isoleucine, acetate, and ß-hydroxybutyrate and decreasing levels of hippurate and fumarate. Several studies have also found a variety of milk metabolites that could be used as indicators of animal health. The ratio of metabolites glycerophosphocholine and phosphocholine found in milk by NMR, for example, has been identified as a biomarker for the risk of ketosis. (Scharen *et al.*, 2021) also explored the relationships between the milk metabolome and cow energy metabolism. The scientists found that indicators like acetone and ß-hydroxybutyrate were highly linked with cows' metabolic condition during early lactation. Xu (2018) investigated the milk metabolome of cows in a negative energy balance state and discovered that the animals' energy balance was substantially linked with various milk metabolites such as glycine, choline, and carnitine. (Tian *et al.*, 2016) also identified a number of milk metabolites that could be used as biomarkers in heat stressed cows, with significant alterations in the milk metabolome of heat stressed cows due to changes in animal metabolism. According to these findings, milk metabolomics could be a useful technique for constant monitoring of herd health.

Metabolomics with Other Technologies: Current Trends in Dairy Research

Metabolomics can help identify the chemical profiles of milk products, but it alone is not enough to fully understand the complex biochemical network involved in milk and milk products. This network includes genes, transcriptions, proteins, and metabolites. To get a better understanding of the changes in metabolism and quality of the product, additional techniques with different biological layers are needed. Multi-omics, which combines metabolomics with other omics technologies such as genomics, metagenomics, transcriptomics, and proteomics, is increasingly being used in milk and milk product research.

One study used a combined metabolomics and proteomics approach to discover reliable milk metabolites for negative energy balance in dairy cattle during lactation. They found that under negative energy balance conditions, proteins associated with lipid metabolism were decreased, while host defense-related proteins were increased. For metabolites, lipids and galactose-1-phosphate were remarkably changed.

Other studies used the joint metabolomics and proteomics technique to identify the role of a specific cattle genotype in milk production and to investigate the effect of mastitis disease on milk microbial and metabolome composition.

They also looked at the metabolomic and metagenomic profiles of milk from cattle with different feeding systems. These studies identified specific metabolites and bacteria families that were correlated with differences in milk from different conditions.

Conclusion and Future Perspectives

In dairy science, metabolomics is a useful tool. Approaches in milk and milk products dealing with various factors from farm to final product dairy demonstrate significant progress made to date and the potential of metabolomics for quality and safety assessment of dairy products in the dairy industry and other research institutions. Metabolomics can be used in dairy breeding programs and milk nutrition initiatives. During milk processing, transportation, and storage, metabolomics can help preserve and improve product quality. Metabolomics-obtained metabolite profiles can also detect chemical or biological contamination in dairy products.

Future metabolomics research may focus on three primary areas. One is evaluating product quality. Seasonal changes cannot be separated from regional origins, diets, dairy animal status, contamination, and other management when producing dairy animals and processing dairy products. Future metabolomics research should examine several elements and their interactions to better reflect the dairy production environment. Second, metabolomics integration with other technologies (multi-omics). The combined omics method (e.g., metabolomics and metagenomics) can provide a better picture of associations and interactions of factors determining dairy product quality (genotypes-phenotypes). Finally, large-scale research uses metabolomics. Dairy products are generated on an industrial scale, yet only laboratory-scale metabolomics investigations have been done. Pilot and industrial metabolomics applications are needed to evaluate dairy product quality. For large-scale simulation, sample collection (within-batch, batch-to-batch, etc.), analysis, and data interpretation may need to be carefully handled. Making decisions in large-scale systems may benefit from statistical quality control (SQC) utilizing a data-driven approach (e.g. process control, acceptance sampling).

These directions and tasks can be accomplished by increasing instrumental analysis techniques in terms of sensitivity and selectivity, and by using artificial intelligence (AI) platforms like machine learning algorithms to manage complicated huge data sets. With these efforts and expertise, metabolomics will assist analyse and improve milk and milk product quality.

References

Carrillo, J. A., He, Y., Li, Y., Liu, J., Erdman, R. A., Sonstegard, T. S., & Song, J. (2016). Integrated metabolomic and transcriptome analyses reveal finishing forage affects metabolic pathways related to beef quality and animal welfare. *Scientific Reports*, *6*(1), 1–16.

Chakraborty, D., Sharma, N., Kour, S., Sodhi, S. S., Gupta, M. K., Lee, S. J., & Son, Y. O. (2022). Applications of omics technology for livestock selection and improvement. *Frontiers in Genetics*, *13*.

Dervishi, E., Reimert, I., van der Zande, L. E., Mathur, P., Knol, E. F., & Plastow, G. S. (2021). Relationship between indirect genetic effects for growth, environmental enrichment, coping style and sex with the serum metabolome profile of pigs. *Scientific Reports*, *11*(1), 23377.

Fontanesi, L. (2016). Metabolomics and livestock genomics: Insights into a phenotyping frontier and its applications in animal breeding. *Animal Frontiers*, *6*(1), 73–79.

Goldansaz, S. A., Guo, A. C., Sajed, T., Steele, M. A., Plastow, G. S., & Wishart, D. S. (2017). Livestock metabolomics and the livestock metabolome: A systematic review. *PloS One*, *12*(5), e0177675.

Guetouache, M., Guessas, B., & Medjekal, S. (2014). Composition and nutritional value of raw milk. *J Issues Biol Sci Pharm Res*, *2350*, 1588.

Hofmann, D. (2017). *The importance of conformational dynamics for drug discovery exemplified with TNFα and AGP1—an NMR study*. ETH Zurich.

Lippa, K. A., Aristizabal-Henao, J. J., Beger, R. D., Bowden, J. A., Broeckling, C., Beecher, C., Clay Davis, W., Dunn, W. B., Flores, R., & Goodacre, R. (2022). Reference materials for MS-based untargeted metabolomics and lipidomics: a review by the metabolomics quality assurance and quality control consortium (mQACC). *Metabolomics*, *18*(4), 24.

Pan, L., Yu, J., Mi, Z., Mo, L., Jin, H., Yao, C., Ren, D., & Menghe, B. (2018). A metabolomics approach uncovers differences between traditional and commercial dairy products in Buryatia (Russian Federation). *Molecules*, *23*(4), 735.

Rocchetti, G., & O'Callaghan, T. F. (2021). Application of metabolomics to assess milk quality and traceability. *Current Opinion in Food Science*, *40*, 168–178.

Sakuma, H., Saito, K., Kohira, K., Ohhashi, F., Shoji, N., & Uemoto, Y. (2017). Estimates of genetic parameters for chemical traits of meat quality in Japanese black cattle. *Animal Science Journal*, *88*(2), 203–212.

Schären, M., Riefke, B., Slopianka, M., Keck, M., Gruendemann, S., Wichard, J., Brunner, N., Klein, S., Snedec, T., & Theinert, K. B. (2021). Aspects of transition cow metabolomics—Part III: Alterations in the metabolome of liver and blood throughout the transition period in cows with different liver metabotypes. *Journal of Dairy Science*, *104*(8), 9245–9262.

Sen, C., Ray, P. R., & Bhattacharyya, M. (2021). A critical review on metabolomic analysis of milk and milk products. *International Journal of Dairy Technology*, *74*(1), 17–31.

Suh, J. H. (2022). Critical review: Metabolomics in dairy science-Evaluation of milk and milk product quality. *Food Research International*, 110984.

Sun, H.-Z., Wang, D.-M., Wang, B., Wang, J.-K., Liu, H.-Y., Guan, L. L., & Liu, J.-X. (2015). Metabolomics of four biofluids from dairy cows: potential biomarkers for milk production and quality. *Journal of Proteome Research*, *14*(2), 1287–1298.

Sundekilde, U. K., Poulsen, N. A., Larsen, L. B., & Bertram, H. C. (2013). Nuclear magnetic resonance metabonomics reveals strong association between milk metabolites and somatic cell count in bovine milk. *Journal of Dairy Science*, *96*(1), 290–299.

Tian, H., Zheng, N., Wang, W., Cheng, J., Li, S., Zhang, Y., & Wang, J. (2016). Integrated metabolomics study of the milk of heat-stressed lactating dairy cows. *Scientific Reports*, *6*(1), 1–10.

Ueda, S., Iwamoto, E., Kato, Y., Shinohara, M., Shirai, Y., & Yamanoue, M. (2019). Comparative metabolomics of Japanese Black cattle beef and other meats using gas chromatography–mass spectrometry. *Bioscience, Biotechnology, and Biochemistry*, *83*(1), 137–147.

Wang, X., & Kadarmideen, H. N. (2020). Metabolite genome-wide association study (mGWAS) and gene-metabolite interaction network analysis reveal potential biomarkers for feed efficiency in pigs. *Metabolites*, *10*(5), 201.

Wu, J., Ye, Y., Quan, J., Ding, R., Wang, X., Zhuang, Z., Zhou, S., Geng, Q., Xu, C., & Hong, L. (2021). Using nontargeted LC-MS metabolomics to identify the Association of Biomarkers in pig feces with feed efficiency. *Porcine Health Management*, *7*(1), 1–10.

Xiao, J. F., Zhou, B., & Ressom, H. W. (2012). Metabolite identification and quantitation in LC-MS/MS-based metabolomics. *TrAC Trends in Analytical Chemistry*, *32*, 1–14.

Xu, W., Vervoort, J., Saccenti, E., van Hoeij, R., Kemp, B., & van Knegsel, A. (2018). Milk metabolomics data reveal the energy balance of individual dairy cows in early lactation. *Scientific Reports*, *8*(1), 1–11.

Yoon, H. S., Cho, C. H., Yun, M. S., Jang, S. J., You, H. J., Kim, J., Han, D., Cha, K. H., Moon, S. H., & Lee, K. (2021). Akkermansia muciniphila secretes a glucagon-like peptide-1-inducing protein that improves glucose homeostasis and ameliorates metabolic disease in mice. *Nature Microbiology*, *6*(5), 563–573.